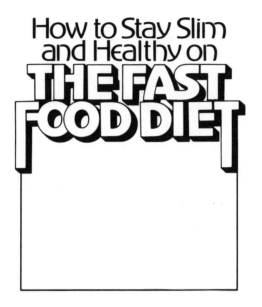

How to Stay Slim and Healthy on THE FAST FOOD DIET

How to Stay Slim and Healthy on THE FAST FOOD DIET

by Judith S. Stern, Sc.D., and R.V. Denenberg

PRENTICE-HALL, INC., *Englewood Cliffs, New Jersey*

ALLEN COUNTY PUBLIC LIBRARY
FORT WAYNE, INDIANA

The Fast Food Diet by Judith S. Stern and R. V. Denenberg
Copyright © 1980 by Judith S. Stern and R. V. Denenberg
All rights reserved. No part of this book may be
reproduced in any form or by any means, except
for the inclusion of brief quotations in a review,
without permission in writing from the publisher.
Address inquiries to Prentice-Hall, Inc., Englewood
Cliffs, N.J. 07632
Printed in the United States of America
Prentice-Hall International, Inc., London
Prentice-Hall of Australia, Pty. Ltd., Sydney
Prentice-Hall of Canada, Ltd., Toronto
Prentice-Hall of India Private Ltd., New Delhi
Prentice-Hall of Japan, Inc., Tokyo
Prentice-Hall of Southeast Asia Pte. Ltd., Singapore
Whitehall Books Limited, Wellington, New Zealand

10   9   8   7   6   5   4   3   2   1

Library of Congress Cataloging in Publicatin Data
Stern, Judith S date
     The fast food diet.

     1. Reducing diets.   2. Restaurants, lunch rooms,
etc.–United States.   I. Denenberg, R. V., date
joint author.   II. Title.
RM222.2.S776   1980   613.2'5   80-10993
ISBN 0-13-307736-5
ISBN 0-13-307738-4 pbk.

Acknowledgements

Writing this book has been, quite literally, a matter of consuming interest to the authors, and we wish to thank our spouses, Tia Schneider Denenberg and Richard C. Stern, for helping us gnaw away at the task. They also offered valuable suggestions in matters of style and substance.

In addition, we acknowledge with gratitude the help of the following persons:

Joan Spaulding, Nancy Yudin, Lillian and Sidney Schneider, Shannon and Dylan Brown, Amanda and Michael Greenwold, Alan Sisitsky, Susan Mackenzie, Irving and Ruth Price, Eric Seidman, Dennis Fawcett.

The authors also thank the restaurant chains that provided us with the nutritional information displayed in the charts in Chapter 7.

Contents

1
INTRODUCTION

Eating fast food is one of those daily rituals of American life, like watching soap operas, that millions of people quietly enjoy while feeling guilty about it.

The enjoyment is not difficult to explain. How many of us can view the many-splendored sight of a triple burger, rising in climactic stages to the sesame seeds, without even a tremor of desire? Who can resist inhaling deeply in that tense, expectant moment when the pizza begins to emerge from the oven, blanketed with—well, you name it.

The guilt is a more complex phenomenon. It probably started, like many other pangs of conscience, with a maternal warning. "Don't eat 'junk' on the way home from school," Mother said. She never specified the consequences, but from then on nameless evils lurked in every forbidden french fry.

Afterward came the many doomed attempts at dieting, each ending abruptly and ingloriously at the drive-in window. You were a three-time non-loser, but in the face of a cheeseburger your defenses were as outflanked as the Maginot Line.

Also, you began hearing that fast food was just "empty calories," bereft of any redeeming nutritional qualities and laced with lethal additives. You kept eating because you liked it, but deep down you began to worry that you might be committing a crime against nature each time you queued up for a chili dog.

This book is intended for you, the guilt-ridden fast food fancier. It presupposes the understandable, inescapable fact that you have a passion for fast food, but it also assumes that you want to be slim and healthy. You can be both, without swearing off all over-the-counter delights, and this book shows you how to do it.

To the health-conscious eater, it offers a careful examination of the nutritional content and quality of fast food and gives suggestions on how to compensate for what may be lacking in the meals that you or the members of

1

your family routinely eat outside the home. To the weight-conscious, it offers a practical plan for incorporating fast food into a sensible, balanced reducing diet on which you can lose up to three pounds a week.

The next chapter assesses the enormous impact that fast food has had on the way all of us eat. Then in Chapter 3 we take a hard look, in the light of the latest scientific data, at the most often-heard claims about the dangers of fast food. A Nutritional Density Score tells you whether you are getting enough vitamins and minerals in fast food (Chapter 4). The most common fast food additives are analyzed and their possible dangers (or benefits) explored in Chapter 5. Chapter 6 describes a step-by-step diet plan that will enable you to lose weight while still eating a satisfying number of meals in fast food restaurants and family-style restaurants.

The Dieter's Guide to Fast Food (Chapter 7) provides a nutritional analysis of the food served at 24 leading chains and offers tips for picking your way among the menus. The guide includes sample whole-day and weekly meal plans that show you how to build in fast food stopovers while keeping your calorie count down and your level of essential nutrients up.

The Fast Food Diet is no miracle cure for obesity, but it is realistic. The "perfect" diet is one that allows you to eat what you want to eat. Trying to lose weight by total deprivation may result in spectacular short-term gains but is rarely successful in the long run. The more you feel deprived of your favorite dishes, the more you fantasize about them. And the more you fantasize, the more likely you are to lapse into uncontrolled binges. Once you start to binge, you satisfy your cravings by overconsumption of prohibited food, so that you may quickly gain back all that you lost in weeks of dieting.

Even if you don't binge, your fantasies may lead you to eat furtively so that no one sees you and so that you don't even remember your secret meals. You go around saying: "Why am I overweight? I never eat anything."

The Fast Food Diet will spare you from Overeater's Amnesia and from fantasies about super burgers, tacos, and fried chicken. If you can't live without fast food, the following pages will tell you how to live with it.

2
THE FAST FOOD PHENOMENON

When President Carter joined three other chiefs of state on the Caribbean island of Guadeloupe for a summit conference in 1978, the catering was put in the skillful hands of Pierre Coffe, a Paris chef who had earned the coveted two-cap rating from a leading French restaurant guide. The President placed his order: hamburgers.

Coffe was dismayed. "You don't ask a two-cap chef for hamburgers," he observed. But in passing up the chance for culinary artistry in favor of the prosaic staple of the drive-ins, the President was merely displaying the attachment to fast food that has become so deeply rooted in most of his fellow countrymen.

The roadside hamburger stand, of course, is at least as old as the automobile. What is new, though, is the explosive growth of national and regional chains of retail outlets offering quick service from a standard, limited menu. Precooked, prepackaged, and automated, fast food has meshed well with American life. Within two decades, it has transformed our eating preferences.

A few statistics demonstrate the fast food industry's extraordinary influence. The United States Senate Subcommittee on Nutrition discovered in 1979 that the typical American adult eats in a fast food outlet nine times a month. Of the nearly 50 million persons who eat out daily, more than a quarter choose fast food. Only 7 percent of American teens and adults manage to avoid eating fast food at least once in six months.

Fast food has become a lucrative, bullish business. There are more than 300 chains, comprising 60,000 outlets. Together they amassed $20 billion in sales in 1978, about a quarter of what Americans spent to feed themselves away from home. No one who reads the chains' record of expansion can doubt that the flame of free enterprise still burns. Many a simple take-out has been transformed in a few years into a multinational corporation. The key financial

3

mechanism is franchising, a system that harnesses the energies and resources of thousands of small businessmen, each profiting from association with the corporate trademark.

The epitome of rapid growth is McDonald's. Now the industry's giant ($4.5 billion is sales in 1978), the chain stemmed from a California restaurant established before World War II. In 1960 there was a chain of 228 McDonald's. By 1970 there were 1,592 outlets. By 1978 that total had more than tripled to 5,185, and McDonald's was operating in 25 foreign countries.

Astonishing amounts of fast food pass under the heat lamps and over the industry's counters. McDonald's adds another billion to its hamburger sale total every few months, consuming a full one percent of the national beef production annually. In a single year, 1978, Kentucky Fried Chicken sold 898 million meals—about four for every inhabitant of the United States.

These prodigious feeding operations have profoundly affected agricultural production and consumption. The humdrum potato had been falling out of favor with the American eater since 1910; but the fast food boom created such an enormous demand for french fries that the use of frozen potatoes, the raw material, soared from 7 pounds per person in 1960 to almost 44 pounds in 1978, according to the U.S. Department of Agriculture. Poultry processors greeted the fast food revolution as eagerly as potato growers, because the fried chicken emporiums helped boost annual demand from 28 to 48 pounds per person during the same period. The doubling of hard cheese consumption—from 8 to 16 pounds per person—was largely the work of pizzaholics, who stimulated the mozzarella market.

Obviously, because of fast food, the American diet is not what it used to be.

Fast food has infiltrated the school lunchroom, once a sanctuary of sober eating, and it has even transformed army chow. "Army cooks can and do sculpture eight different approved edges for pie crust and cook potatoes in a dozen different ways," military affairs analyst Drew Middleton has commented, "but the serviceman is likely to head for the counter that provides cheeseburgers, tacos, french fries, and fried chicken."

To keep pace, the Defense Department has commissioned the successor to the chuck wagon: a mobile burger stand. Fast food technology helped the army abolish the venerable canned C-ration—more dreaded than the enemy—in favor of the foil-wrapped MRE (Meal Ready to Eat), which is heated in the pouch. Crunchier french fries may even boost reenlistments.

Americans' devotion to fast food has been matched abroad. Along with jazz, fast food is a vehicle for the export of American culture, although sometimes other nations have been quick to adopt the innovation as their own. That was demonstrated when Japanese boy scouts touring the United States were asked by a Chicago newsman what surprised them most about this country. "I didn't know they had McDonald's here, too," one scout replied.

Indeed, the avenues of Japan are lined with Golden Arches and the familiar symbols of Dunkin' Donuts, Pizza Hut, and Dairy Queen—with subtitles in Japanese and, as is the custom of that country, plastic models or photographs of the burgers and cones to help the patrons order. These and other chains have carried the flag—and an order of fries—to such far-flung outposts as the Persian Gulf sheikdoms and the Pacific islands.

Fast food even crosses ideological lines. In 1979 the People's Republic of China dispatched a delegation to study American fast food methods so that workers could be fed more quickly. It takes so long to prepare meals in China that factory lunch hours drag on, cutting into production time. The Chinese have already begun a campaign to wean their people away from noodles and toward the easier-to-serve carbohydrate, bread—possibly the first step on the way to burger buns and sandwiches.

Fortunately, the proper beverage is at hand. Occidental soft drinks have been introduced, their marketing aided by the happy coincidence that the words Coca-Cola roughly approximate the Chinese phrase for "tasty." No one is quite sure, however, whether "finger lickin' good" will mean much to a nation that uses chopsticks.

Some Europeans, like the Parisian chef who served the President, evidently view fast food as an invasion by gastronomic barbarism, but others look upon it with the same sense of deliverance that they felt on D-Day. Complaining of the poor restaurant food in England, a letter to *The Guardian,* a London newspaper, asked, "Isn't it about time we had the proper equivalent of the American fast-food joint?"

Americans respond with chauvinistic pride in fast food, considering it an edible manifestation of Yankee ingenuity. When a British conglomerate purchased the Howard Johnson chain in 1979, Senator John Tower denounced the sale in broad Texas hyperbole as "blatant foreign economic adventurism . . . almost more than ice-cream-loving red-blooded Americans can take." He trumpeted the modern equivalent of Fifty-four Forty or Fight: "Wake up, America! Colonel Sanders, Pizza Hut, and Taco Bell may be next."

What accounts for the success of fast food? Sheer affluence is apparently a large factor. American families—especially the increasing number with working mothers—have more money to eat out and more reason to do so. The proportion of the average family food budget devoted to eating out has been rising steadily. It is now about one-third, and within the 1980's the amount spent eating out is expected to equal the amount spent on home cooking.

Much of that mealtime money finds its way into the registers of the chains, possibly because fast food offers instant gratification. It earns its name not only because it can be prepared fast and served fast, but also because it can be eaten fast—virtually inhaled. Fast food is also portable and usually requires only one hand, which means that even more time can be saved by one's eating it while driving or working.

Speed has been achieved through mass production. The food rolls off the assembly line like Fords in Detroit. Consider this description of how one chain manufactures burgers:

After the beef undergoes a final grind, it is transferred in stainless steel buckets and loaded into Formax machines. The sophisticated machine forms patties at the rate of 540 per minute with precise control over weight, shape and size. The hamburgers are then frozen at precisely controlled temperatures.

Given this uniformity, obviously no burger will ever reach epicurean heights. There is not much room in the process for *je ne sais quois.* But the other side of the coin is that no burger will be an unexpected disaster. The virtue of standardization is that, for better or worse, the customer knows what he or she is getting and what it will cost. The cost, moreover, is relatively modest. The average price of a restaurant meal in 1978 was almost $7. The average fast food meal was less than $3, and there was usually no tip. (The next year a few chains actually lowered some prices as an anti-inflationary gesture.)

Some connoisseurs deride the notion that fast food tastes good, but no less a gourmet than Craig Claiborne, *The New York Times* food critic and a cookbook author, has sampled a chain-produced burger and pronounced it "quite swallowable" with a "highly compatible onion flavor." Most of us are less demanding. Besides, the fast food industry helped create the tastes in food that it now satisfies.

The archetype of fast food is the burger. Its origins have been traced to medieval Europe, where it was apparently a dish of raw meat, shredded with a knife. It became quite popular along the Baltic coast, including the German port city of Hamburg, as a change of pace from the usual herring snack. German immigrants carried the dish with them to St. Louis. At the World's Fair there in 1904, it was sold cooked by vendors. But the meatball-shaped Baltic burger needed one technological improvement to adapt it to American life: it had to be flattened to make it fry more evenly.

Building upon established favorites like burgers and hot dogs, the fast food industry cultivated a wide following for other dishes, like pizza, that had been confined to a single ethnic group or region. Eaters who formerly could not tell a burrito from a beachball are now patronizing taco stands thousands of miles from the Rio Grande. Fast food restaurants are helping to popularize "natural food." At the Sunflower Drive-In near Sacramento, California, for example, you can order a meatless Super Nutburger on whole grain bun with an order of falafel and wash it down with a glass of raw buttermilk. There are even fast food chains that serve nothing but baked potatoes.

The industry's effective salesmanship is in part a triumph of advertising, particularly saturation of the airwaves. The message has gotten across. As

Senator George McGovern, chairman of the Nutrition Subcommittee, wistfully noted, "Ronald McDonald, McDonald's corporate symbol, is so prominently advertised that in a 1972 survey, 96 percent of all U.S. schoolchildren could identify this clown character, an enviable achievement [that] any politician in this country, I am sure, would like to duplicate."

The industry has also correctly gauged the national passion for conspicuous sanitation. Bright lighting and cheerily colored plastic counters create an antiseptic aura, maintained by diligent company inspectors. The dirty dish problem has been eliminated by encapsulating food in paper or plastic containers, a serving method eminently suited to the no-deposit nation. Wendy's, a national chain, reported in 1979 that the french fry containers it used in a year, if laid end to end, would cover the distance between New York and Los Angeles more than ten times.

Paper packaging is conducive to mobility, another fast food success factor. White Castle, a precursor of the quick-service movement, opened its first burger stand in 1921 (price: 5 cents); but the industry's main burst of expansion occurred much later. It happened along the arteries of the burgeoning mid-century suburbs, where the car was also the family dining room, and along the cloverleaves of the Interstate Highway System. Once the taste for fast food became well entrenched, the chains followed the suburban commuter to work in the city center.

They have not always been welcome neighbors, because of the crowds the outlets attract and because the typical building design owes more to the principles of brand identification than to architecture. One community, Edgartown, Massachusetts, has gone so far as to ban large fast food restaurants, defined as those having more than one take-out window and six parking spaces.

Zoning laws are unlikely to stem the tide if it is true, as some have argued, that fast food satisfies deep-seated psychological needs. *Natural History* magazine has suggested that eating fast food is a quasi-religious ritual involving "temporary subordination of individual differences in a social and cultural collectivity.... [N]ot only do we communicate that we are hungry, enjoy hamburgers, and have inexpensive tastes but also that we are willing to adhere to a value system and a series of behaviors dictated by an exterior entity. In a land of tremendous ethnic, social, economic, and religious diversity, we proclaim that we share something with millions of other Americans."

To other psychological analysts, the American attachment to fast food represents a yearning for something one can depend upon, something reliable and honest. Since burgers coming off a conveyor belt are standard and don't pretend to be anything more than they are, they are never a disappointment. In the age of modest expectations, fast food is the perfect sustenance.

Yet for a nation that has made fast food part of its lifestyle, we are curiously ambivalent about eating it. We vote with our feet—or our mouths—by lining up at the counters. The sales figures are undeniable proof of popular esteem. But all the same, fast food is often deprecated, spoken of as nutritionally decadent at best and possibly hazardous to health.

Just how "nutritious" is fast food? The next chapter examines this controversial subject.

3
WHAT'S WRONG (OR RIGHT) WITH FAST FOOD?

Testifying before the Senate in 1979, a representative of the fast food industry complained that "We have . . . had to suffer the ridicule and the abuse of the bureaucratic regulators who look at our industry as junk food purveyors and merchants of empty calories" even though "our industry can provide good nutrition as readily, if not more readily, than our chief competitor, the homemaker."

The allegations to which he alluded are certainly heard often. The question is whether the charges have a basis in fact or whether the industry, as the representative implied, cooks as well as Mother but has been victimized by sheer prejudice. In this chapter we assess the claims made by the industry's detractors about the effects of eating fast food.

These are the major claims:

CLAIM: FAST FOOD MAKES YOU OVERWEIGHT

Paradoxically, a major defect in fast food is not that it is non-nutritious but that it is too nutritious, at least in the sense that it helps overfulfill our daily quota of calories. Calories represent the energy in food that our bodies burn up. As a nation, we tend to end each day with a surplus of energy intake over energy expenditures. That wasn't always the case. At the beginning of the century Americans ate even more calories than we do now and were leaner. But the pre-automotive, pretelephonic age, when many people wielded axes and hoes, required a good deal of physical effort. Today we have become much more sedentary. For some, virtually the only rapid, sustained bodily motion is the movement of the hands bringing food to the mouth.

As a result, although famine may stalk much of the world, America's most common nutritional disorder is just the reverse—overeating. Obesity, in fact, has reached epidemic proportions.

9

The number of overweight Americans is uncertain, but studies suggest that up to 80 million persons (as much as 40 percent of the adult population) could be so classified. The trend toward obesity begins, disturbingly, in childhood and adolescence, and the evidence suggests that such youngsters do not lose their "baby fat" but rather go on to become fat adults. The odds against a fat 12-year-old slimming down later are 4 to 1; they rise to 28 to 1 if the excess poundage hasn't been shed by the end of adolescence.

Obesity progresses with age. A typical 5-foot, 4-inch woman, for example, is likely to distend her figure by adding 15 to 25 additional pounds between the ages of 25 and 55. (To compensate for our lack of girth control, the seats in the new Metropolitan Opera House that opened in New York City in the 1960's had to be made two inches wider than those in the old opera house.)

Overweight persons not only suffer social embarrassment and discrimination in the work place but incur some risk of serious illness and shortened life span. The list of conditions to which the obese are more susceptible reads like the index to a textbook on killer diseases. They include cardiovascular and cerebrovascular disease, diabetes, hypertension, angina, and gallbladder and lung dysfunctions. The obese are also more likely to suffer complications in surgery.

How do fast foods contribute to the obesity menace? For one thing, they certainly make eating easier. We are led down a primrose path lined with inviting, convenient eateries. Almost everywhere we turn—at work, at school, at play—we find ourselves near a take-out window. The outlets, after all, have been strategically placed to be where we are. So unless we are careful, our calorie intake can be augmented quite insidiously. In some ways, it is the nutritional equivalent of impulse buying.

Fast food, moreover, tends to be calorically dense, so that in a typical meal we get a disproportionately large share of our daily needs. How great are these needs? Listed on page 11 are the number of calories that persons of various ages require each 24-hour period to maintain their weights, assuming they perform only light physical activity, such as occasionally walking to the office water cooler. (Caloric needs decrease with age because of metabolic changes.)

Now consider the number of calories in two typical fast food meals:

Chicken dinner (3 pieces of chicken,
mashed potatoes with gravy, and roll)
12-ounce soft drink

TOTAL CALORIES 1,100

Super burger (with everything)
Large order of french fries
Chocolate shake

TOTAL CALORIES 1,230

Body Weight (lb)	Age				
	22	35	45	55	65
MEN	Calories Daily				
110	2,200	2,100	2,000	1,950	1,850
121	2,350	2,250	2,150	2,100	1,950
132	2,500	2,400	2,300	2,250	2,100
143	2,650	2,500	2,400	2,350	2,200
154	2,800	2,650	2,600	2,500	2,400
165	2,950	2,800	2,700	2,650	2,500
176	3,050	2,900	2,800	2,700	2,600
187	3,200	3,050	2,950	2,850	2,700
198	3,350	3,200	3,100	3,000	2,800
209	3,500	3,400	3,200	3,100	2,900
220	3,700	3,500	3,400	3,300	3,100
WOMEN					
88	1,550	1,450	1,450	1,400	1,300
99	1,700	1,600	1,550	1,500	1,450
110	1,800	1,700	1,650	1,600	1,500
121	1,950	1,850	1,800	1,750	1,650
128	2,000	1,900	1,850	1,800	1,700
132	2,050	1,950	1,900	1,800	1,700
143	2,200	2,100	2,000	1,950	1,850
154	2,300	2,200	2,100	2,050	1,950

Note: Reprinted from the 1968 RDAs with permission from the National Academy of Sciences.

If the eater were a 35-year-old man weighing 154 pounds, either meal would satisfy about 45 percent of his daily calorie needs. For a 128-pound woman of the same age, the chicken meal would represent 58 percent of her calorie allotment for the day and the burger meal 65 percent. That's without dessert.

The calorie overload tends to be even greater because fast food is indeed eaten fast. Rapid eating, some studies have shown, results in your eating more than if you just munched and chewed at a leisurely pace, perhaps waiting 20 minutes in between courses. The reason is that it takes a while for the satiety sensors in the brain to realize that your stomach is filling up. By the time you feel satisfied, you probably have had another burger that you wouldn't have missed had you eaten slowly. So the actual meal eaten may be much larger and use up an even greater share of the daily calorie quota than the examples above.

Fixed portion sizes are another fattening influence. All restaurant food tends to come in portions designed to satisfy the appetite of a large, ravenous customer. Smaller, less hungry patrons could do with less, but if it's put on the plate most of us will eat it. (Think of the starving children in other countries, your parents said.) Fast food outlets usually adhere to this practice, and they make it even worse by using large size as a marketing strategy. Plain burgers pale into insignificance beside jumbo, super-special, colossal, and double-decker constructions. The very names subliminally associate bigness with goodness. In contrast, few of us are likely to be overawed by the prospect of consuming something called, say, a Midget Burger.

A few chains, however, have adopted the encouraging policy of offering "junior" portions. Whether or not intended only for the kids, they do offer an opportunity to limit our eating without having to pay for wasted food.

Of course, a fast food meal by itself would not be fattening if nothing else were eaten that day. No single meal, in that sense, is likely to be a caloric disaster. But the fast food meal requires the remaining calorie intake to be rigidly controlled. It's difficult. Getting most of your food energy in one sitting does not leave much flexibility for making it through the rest of the day. But it can be done, and in Chapter 7 you will see how.

CLAIM: FAST FOOD DOES NOT HAVE ENOUGH PROTEIN

Americans suffer from a strange obsession, which might be called the Protein Fetish. We seem haunted by the fear that we are not getting enough protein, and any food product that conceivably can be called "high protein" or "protein enriched" seems to do better in the marketplace.

There are many reasons for this obsession. Some people consider protein "healthier" than other constituents of food, and they labor under the impression that if some is good, more must be better. Protein is valued by body-builders, for example, who mistakenly think that large amounts will help them expand their biceps. Eating animal protein seems to increase with affluence, as a kind of status symbol, because it is a relatively expensive food. It may also have other symbolic value. Most of our protein comes from eating meat, and nutritionist Jean Mayer has argued that the "more men sit at their desks, the more they need reassurance of their maleness by eating red meat. It is the motorcycle of the middle-aged."

Protein, of course, is a vital nutrient, supplying raw materials (called amino acids) that our bodies need to build tissue. However, the American population consumes much more protein than it needs for proper nutrition. The Food and Nutrition Board of the National Academy of Sciences, which determines the Recommended Dietary Allowance (RDA) of each nutrient, has set the daily protein figure at 56 grams (about 2 ounces) for an adult man and 44 grams for an adult woman. That figure is considered to be a generous overestimate. (Faced with the task of feeding the whole world, the United Nations Food and Agriculture Organization had decided that a person could get by nicely which much less, perhaps two-thirds of the RDA.) Yet the average

American tends to consume about twice the recommended amount. The U.S. Agriculture Department reported daily protein consumption for the population as a whole at 104 grams per person in 1976.

Fast food, if anything, encourages protein overconsumption. Most of the meals are rich in protein foods. A super burger would provide 25.6 grams of protein, or about 46 percent of the man's and 56 percent of the woman's daily needs. Even a pizza makes a sizable contribution to one's protein supply. Two slices of a modest (13-inch) cheese pizza supplies 24 grams, and the total would increase dramatically if a more elaborate topping (more cheese, pepperoni sausage) were added.

Is overconsumption of protein hazardous? If you're a healthy adult, there is little evidence of danger in overconsuming protein as long as you don't displace other essential nutrients, especially carbohydrates, and don't over-consume fat. Excess protein simply will be burned up as food energy or stored as fat. However, it is a rather wasteful use of your food dollar. The same calories could be obtained much more cheaply from carbohydrates.

Ecological concerns about protein consumption are often expressed. Some environmentalists object to the use of energy and grain to produce an excess amount of animal protein. Today, though, only 25 percent of livestock food is grain; the remaining 75 percent comes from plant roughage and by-products that would not be available to us as food unless it were converted into meat by animals.

CLAIM: FAST FOOD HAS TOO MUCH FAT

Many fast foods are undeniably high in fat. A typical chicken dinner or a fish sandwich and fries each provide about 50 percent of their calories in the form of fat. Such large proportions significantly abet the national trend toward a high-fat diet.

Fat consumption has risen sharply since the beginning of the century, when it represented about 30 percent of the caloric intake. Today it represents about 40 percent. What is wrong with that? For one thing, high fat consumption encourages obesity, because even though both fats and carbohydrates are made up of the same constituents—carbon, hydrogen, and oxygen—fat is a much more densely packed repository of food energy. A single gram of fat contains more than twice as many calories as a gram of carbohydrate or protein, 9 compared to 4. So fat-laden food makes a calorie surplus more likely. As an example, a five-ounce baked potato would supply about 106 calories, but if you eat less than three ounces of french fries instead, you take in 172 calories.

Another important reason for concern about the high fat level is that it is strongly associated with the condition that causes half the deaths in the United States each year—heart disease. The exact relationship is complex and subject to controversy, but many experts agree with this scenario: Cholesterol a waxy substance, is deposited on the inner lining of the arteries, impeding the flow of blood or causing the formation of clots that can ultimately block an artery. The result is a heart attack or a stroke.

The obvious strategy is to reduce cholesterol; this can partly be accomplished by limiting one's intake of dietary cholesterol contained in food such as egg yolks. (The Senate Nutrition Subcommittee has recommended restricting cholesterol intake to 300 mg* a day.) But the body manufactures its own cholesterol, because it is a necessary constituent of the membranes that surround each of our cells. A person may go on producing enough to have excessive blood levels of cholesterol even if he or she eats very little dietary cholesterol. Some of the raw materials for the production process are the fats, particularly saturated fats. They permeate meats like beef and pork (even when the meat has been stripped of visible fat) and dairy products such as butter, cream, and cheese. A low-fat diet, therefore, can help to lower your blood cholesterol.

For that reason, the Senate Nutrition Subcommittee recommended reducing the overall level of fat consumption to 30 percent of calories, where it stood at the beginning of the century. The Committee also urged that the proportion of saturated fat in our diet be lowered so that only 10 percent of the caloric intake is saturated fat. The remaining 20 percent fat would be mono-unsaturated fats, which seem not to assist cholesterol production, and polyunsaturated fats, which actively lower blood cholesterol. Mono-unsaturated and polyunsaturated fats are produced mainly by plants. They differ in their chemical structure from the saturated fats.

Not everyone accepts this scenario, and some argue that the Senate's prescription amounts to a therapeutic diet for which normally healthy people have no need. But since large amounts of fat in the diet do not have any obvious benefits, it seems prudent to try to modify our eating patterns.

What's more, there is also some evidence, although still highly speculative, of a connection between high fat intake, especially of animal fat, and another disease: cancer. The deputy director of the National Cancer Institute, Dr. Gio Gori, testified in 1976 that "as the dietary intake of fat increases, you have an almost linear [one-for-one] increase in the incidence of breast and colon cancer." The supposed connection is based largely upon population studies, and the mechanism by which fat might be related to cancer is not yet known.

How can we limit our fat intake? Primarily by eating less meat and leaner meats, cutting off all visible fat, eating more poultry, seafood, grains, fruits, and vegetables, and using less fat and oils in our cooking. To help limit your fat intake when eating fast foods, check the fat content of specific menu items in Chapter 7.

*mg = milligrams. One milligram is one-thousandth of a gram.

CLAIM: FAST FOOD IS TOO HIGH IN SUGAR

Although fast food "main dishes" themselves are generally not high in sugar, they are surrounded by an array of shakes, colas, sundaes, and desserts that may contain very little else. A 12-ounce cola, for example, provides 150 calories. If four of these a day are drunk, a person might imbibe a quarter to a third of his or her calories in the form of sugar. Soft drink consumption, moreover, has been on the increase. Americans downed 493 8-ounce servings per capita in 1976, compared to only 192 servings in 1960. (There are also some incidental high-sugar items—ketchup has about 20 percent sugar—but unless you are in the habit of drowning all your food in ketchup, you probably would not ingest enough to notice the difference.)

What's wrong with high sugar intake? If anything deserves the term "empty calories," it is refined sugar. Sugar is 99.9 percent pure sucrose, in crystalline form. It provides energy but is totally bereft of vitamins, minerals, and other nutrients. The lack of these redeeming qualities is not especially serious if sugar is used in moderation as a flavor enhancer, but it *is* serious if sugar becomes a significant portion of a person's diet, displacing calories that might bring valuable nutrients with them.

Although many people are convinced that "sugar makes you fat," there is no evidence that obese persons consume a higher proportion of sugar than do the nonobese. The hazards lie elsewhere. Sugar is responsible for an epidemic of tooth decay. Bacteria in the mouth convert sugar into an acid that causes cavities; the process is especially effective if the sugar is gooey and sticks well to the teeth. For a small number of people, sugar is implicated in heart disease. Large amounts of it can cause high levels of fat (triglycerides) in the blood, a cardiac risk factor. Finally, there is evidence that persons with a family history suggesting predisposition to diabetes would be wise to curtail their sugar intake.

The national penchant for sweet-tasting foods, which causes high sugar use, also stimulates the demand for artificial sweeteners. Their dangers are now much debated (see Chapter 5).

CLAIM: FAST FOOD CONTAINS TOO LITTLE FIBER

The increased intake of refined sugar and meat has displaced from our diet the complex carbohydrates—the starches contained in grains, peas, beans, lentils, and other vegetables. Not only has this deprived us of some of the nutrients that are found along with complex carbohydrates, but it has also robbed our diet of much of its fiber content, what Grandma called "roughage."

Fiber is found only in foods of plant origin. Highly refined food contains less fiber than whole-grain products. Sugar is devoid of fiber. There are various types of fiber, each having a characteristic effect. Bran fiber, for example, acts as a laxative. Pectin, another type, helps to reduce blood cholesterol.

Until recently fiber was pretty much ignored by nutritionists. Now its role in our diet is being reexamined because studies have shown that in areas of the world where the diet is rich in fiber, such as rural Africa, the incidence of diseases like cancer of the colon and heart disease is lower than in countries like the United States, where people eat very little fiber. While fiber is not a cure-all—no one nutrient is—increasing the amount of fiber in your diet may not only help to lower your cholesterol level but could also prevent or ameliorate hemorrhoids. Fiber is also the treatment of choice for diverticulitis (a ballooning and inflammation of the intestinal wall, which is common in middle age).

Although the experts do not quite agree on how much fiber the American diet should include, they do agree that Americans eat too little—less than 5 grams per day. Fast food contributes to a low fiber level, because it has only tiny amounts. A special burger offers but 0.7 grams of fiber, a shake none. Even a large order of french fries contains a mere 0.6 grams. Someone who made a lunch of two slices of a 10-inch cheese pizza plus a cola would get 1.3 grams for the meal. If a person requiring, say, 1,900 calories for the day made up the total with meals containing that level of fiber, the whole day's eating would yield only 3.1 grams.

Obviously, a habitual fast food eater needs to balance the rest of his or her intake carefully to ensure getting a reasonable amount of fiber. Eating whole-grain cereals for breakfast, plus fruits and vegetables, will increase the fiber in your diet. (See the meal plans in Chapter 7.)

CLAIM: FAST FOOD HAS TOO MUCH SODIUM

Sodium is a necessary nutrient, but present-day eaters simply overdo it. The latest Recommended Dietary Allowance is 1.1 to 3 grams of sodium daily, yet the average American soaks up from 6 to 18 grams. (Table salt is 40 percent sodium.) That huge excess may represent a significant health hazard to some, because high sodium levels are suspected of being a cause or at least a factor contributing to the incidence of high blood pressure (hypertension), a disease that afflicts well over 25 million people in this country.

The evidence for the link between sodium intake and hypertension is indirect. There are three bits of evidence.

First, in laboratory rats that are genetically susceptible to hypertension, high sodium intake induces the condition. However, only about 15 to 20 percent of Americans are similarly susceptible to inherited hypertension.

Second, in countries like Japan, where sodium intake is very high, the incidence of hypertension is two to four times that of the United States.

Third, in hypertensive individuals, blood pressure drops when sodium intake drops.

But other key pieces of information are lacking. In particular, we still do not know whether a high sodium intake in childhood or adolescence will make one more likely to become hypertensive in later years or whether restricting sodium levels while young prevents the condition from developing.

Against this background, the Senate Nutrition Subcommittee urged reduction in sodium intake to a maximum of two grams (2,000 mg) a day, the equivalent of about a teaspoonful of salt. But that is easier said than done. Even if you threw away your salt shaker, you would still get more sodium than you need from processed foods, like fast foods, which rely heavily on salt to perk up the flavor. Even condiments like ketchup and pickles are heavily salted. (Two round pickle slices harbor 186 mg.)

The sodium content in fast food varies considerably from dish to dish and from chain to chain. Here are the ranges for some typical items:

	Sodium Content in mg
Super burgers	708 to 1,083
Pizza (13-inch, two slices)	800 to 1,400
Fried chicken dinner	1,915 to 2,285
Fish sandwich	421 to 837
Taco	79 to 460
Shake	250 to 300

There are some ways of exercising individual discretion, however, so as to make a big difference in sodium intake. For example, ten french fries with salt and a tablespoon of ketchup add up to about 370 mg of sodium, almost 20 percent of the daily allowance recommended by the Nutrition Subcommittee. If you leave off the salt and the ketchup, the same french fries would give you only 2 mg, which should help you get through the day without a sodium overdose.

CLAIM: FAST FOODS CAUSE GAS

Scientists are still debating the causes of intestinal gas or flatus. Apparently there are two sources. One is swallowed air. The other is the action of bacteria in the large intestine upon certain nondigestible carbohydrates contained in vegetables such as beans. In one study, when subjects ate 57 percent of their calories in the form of pork and beans, the amount of gas generated was more than four times greater than normal.

Extremely flatugenic (gas-inducing) foods include milk, onions, celery, carrots, raisins, bananas, apricots, prune juice, pretzels, bagels, wheat germ, and brussels sprouts. Among the moderately flatugenic foods are pastries, potatoes, eggplant, citrus fruits, apples, and bread. With the exception of some Mexican food, fast foods are less gas-inducing than most other foods in our diet.

4
THE NUTRIENT DENSITY SCORE: MEASURING VITAMINS AND MINERALS

Unless you are one of those pill-poppers who is content to get vitamins and minerals from a bottle, you rely on food to supply them. That's more sensible, in any event, because scientific understanding of the body's requirements is imperfect. No one can be confident that pills have it all. But we do know that eating a balanced diet can meet your needs.

For that reason, the doubts that are sometimes raised about the vitamin and mineral adequacy of fast food ought to give pause to anyone who regularly gratifies his yearning for triple-decker super deluxes. Are those meals just a lot of idle chewing and swallowing? The fast food fancier should ascertain whether his favorites are low in vitamins and minerals, or whether they supply enough of his needs for those nutrients to beat the "junk food" reputation.

How low is low? How much is enough? That, like our protein and calorie requirements, has been determined by the Food and Nutrition Board of the National Academy of Sciences. The Board's Recommended Dietary Allowances (RDAs), updated most recently in 1979, include ten vitamins and six minerals. (There are also provisional recommendations for twelve other nutrients for which the amounts needed have not been established precisely.)

The daily allowances vary according to a person's age, sex, and body weight. For some nutrients, the allowances are so microscopic that they are measured in micrograms. A microgram, abbreviated μg is one-thousandth of a milligram. (As a point of reference, the average green pea weighs 430 milligrams.) Other nutrients, because they come in various chemical forms, are measured not by weight but by a standard measure of biological activity, called International Units. Here are the RDAs for a typical woman between the ages of 23 and 50.

Vitamin A: 4,000 International Units
Vitamin D: 250 International Units or 5 mg

19

Vitamin E: 8 mg
Vitamin C: 60 mg
Thiamin or vitamin B_1 : 1 mg
Riboflavin or vitamin B_2 : 1.2 mg
Niacin: 13 mg
Vitamin B_6 : 2 mg
Folacin: 400 μg
Vitamin B_{12} : 3 μg
Calcium: 800 mg
Phosphorus: 800 mg
Magnesium: 300 mg
Iron: 18 mg
Zinc: 15 mg
Iodine: 150 μg

These are the provisional recommendations:

Vitamin K: 70 to 140 μg
Biotin: 100 to 200 μg
Pantothenic acid: 4 to 7 mg
Copper: 2 to 3 mg
Manganese: 2.5 to 5 mg
Fluoride: 1.5 to 4 mg
Chromium: 0.05 to 0.2 mg
Selenium: 0.05 to 0.2 mg
Molybdenum: 0.15 to 0.5 mg
Sodium: 1,100 to 3,300 mg
Potassium: 1,875 to 5,625 mg
Chloride: 1,700 to 5,100 mg

Although vitamins and minerals are needed in tiny amounts, their absence makes a crucial difference, because they are essential for sustaining metabolism and, in the case of calcium and phosphorus, forming structural components such as bone. Long-term deprivation results in deficiency diseases with serious symptoms. These are some of the conditions that may develop:

Vitamins

Vitamin A: Night blindness; scarring of the cornea; eventual blindness; scaly skin; infections of eye, nasal passages, sinuses, ear, lungs, genitourinary tract.
Vitamin B_1 : Beriberi: mental confusion; painful calf muscles; peripheral paralysis; edema or muscle wasting; enlarged heart; eventual cardiac failure.

Vitamin B₂ : Fissures at the corners of the mouth; sore tongue and mouth; sensitivity to light, weakness.

Vitamin B₆ : Weakness; anemia; ataxia; abdominal pain; seizures.

Vitamin B₁₂ : Pernicious anemia; numbness of legs.

Vitamin C: Scurvy: red, swollen, and bleeding gums; poor wound healing; swelling of joints; anemia; poor bone and tooth development.

Vitamin E: Increased fragility of red blood cells.

Folacin: Anemia; gastrointestinal disturbances; depression; nervousness; fatigue; weakness.

Niacin: Pellagra: dermatitis; diarrhea; mental confusion; eventually delirium.

Pantothenic Acid: Abdominal pains; cramping pains in arms and legs; burning sensations of feet; apathy; lethargy.

Minerals

Calcium: Stunting of growth; poor quality of bones and teeth; rickets; osteoporosis.

Chromium: Impaired glucose tolerance; (suspected) atherosclerosis.

Copper: Anemia; depigmentation.

Fluoride: Increased number of dental caries.

Iodine: Goiter: undue sensitivity to cold; thickening and drying of skin; loss of hair; anemia; slowing of physical and mental reactions; if deficiency occurs during first three months of pregnancy, severe mental retardation of child.

Iron: Anemia.

Magnesium: Delirium; depression; weakness; tremors; vertigo; tetany. (Alcoholics often deficient.)

Manganese: In animals: failure to grow, sterility.

Molybdenum: Weak and malformed young animals.

Phosphorus: Weakness; bone pain; demineralization of bone; loss of calcium.

Selenium: Poor growth; liver damage.

Zinc: Hypogeusia (loss of sense of taste); in children and adolescents: poor growth and delayed sexual development.

Does fast food contribute its share of the vitamins and minerals needed to prevent deficiency? The vitamin and mineral "adequacy" of fast foods varies, depending on who eats them. As an example, let's take a 20-year-old man who requires 2,900 calories per day and a 35-year-old woman who needs only 1,900 calories. Their requirement for magnesium is almost the same, 300 mg per day for the woman, 350 for the man. That means if the man ate a super burger, a regular order of fries, and a vanilla shake (about 1,060 calories and 97 mg of magnesium), he would get 37 percent of his day's calorie quota and 28 percent of his magnesium. For him, that's almost adequate magnesium for the meal. A woman eating the identical meal would be getting 32 percent of her RDA for magnesium, but she would be taking in 56 percent of her calories. That's too little magnesium, considering the large portion of calories. At this rate, she would have to exceed greatly her calorie quota to get enough magnesium for the day.

The contrast between the man and the woman is even more extreme in the case of the nutrient iron. The man's intake of iron ideally should be 10 mg per day, the woman's 18 mg. The 4.9 mg of iron that the burger meal provides would satisfy 49 percent of his daily iron quota (a good nutritional buy) but only 27 percent of hers. It would be virtually impossible for the woman to meet her day's need for iron in the remaining 840 calories, unless she ate a very rich source of iron, like liver.

Using this approach, we can determine the vitamin and mineral adequacy of fast food by calculating what we shall call its Nutrient Density Score (NDS). The score for any nutrient in a meal is found by dividing the percentage of the RDA supplied by the food by the percentage of the daily calories supplied, and multiplying by 100. An NDS of 100 means a good return on the caloric investment. If it's more than 100, it's a superior deal from a nutritional standpoint.

Take the example of the man and woman and the super burger meal. In his meal, the NDS for magnesium is 76 and for iron 132. For her the identical meal would produce scores of 57 and 48 respectively—well below the ideal of 100 or more.

Fast food meals will be evaluated here as if they were for that 35-year old woman who needs 1,900 calories each day to maintain her weight. It makes sense to do so since fast food presents special difficulties for women because of their relatively low calorie needs. Many nutrients must be squeezed into few calories. Also, dieters are chiefly women—65 percent of women go on at least one diet each year—and the reduced calorie intake makes it even more important to pay attention to nutrient density.

Tastes and menus vary, of course, but the following four meals are representative:

1. Super burger, regular order of french fries, vanilla shake.
2. Fried chicken (three pieces), roll, cole slaw, potatoes.
3. Half of 10-inch cheese pizza, iced tea with two teaspoons of sugar.
4. Fried fish sandwich, regular order of french fries, vanilla shake.

Let's look first at the vitamin content, then the mineral content, of these meals.

VITAMINS

The four fast food meals are a good source of vitamin B_1 (thiamin)—although the chicken meal is lower in thiamin—B_2 (riboflavin), B_{12}, and niacin. (If fortified milk products were consumed, the meals would also be adequate for children's needs for vitamin D; adults usually get all they need from sunshine.) The meals tend to be low in vitamins A, B_6, C, folacin, and pantothenic acid. But with appropriate food choices for the rest of your day, the proper levels can be reached. The chart gives the details.

Vitamin A (retinol)

Fast foods in general are low in vitamin A. Our fish menu, for example, provides 52 percent of a woman's calories and only 15 percent of vitamin A (NDS = 30). The NDS for both the burger and chicken menus is 36. The pizza faired the best (NDS = 72).

How can you make up for the lack of vitamin A in fast foods? The key is to eat green and yellow vegetables (broccoli, carrots, squash) in your other meals. If a fast food chain has a salad bar, taking advantage of the carrots, tomatoes, and even lettuce will add significantly to your A quota.

Vitamin B_1 (thiamin)

Thiamin is present in many foods, with the notable exception of pure sugar and fat; that fact is reflected in the four meals. The NDS for the burger, pizza, and fish meals is over 100, and the chicken meal scores almost 75. Good sources of thiamin in the meals include the enriched flour in the pizza dough and rolls, the relatively lean burger beef, and the poultry. At this rate, there's not much need to worry about your thiamin quota for the rest of the day.

Vitamin B_2 (riboflavin)

All the menus are excellent sources of riboflavin. The burger, pizza, and fish meals outdo themselves with scores of over 125, and even the low scorer, the chicken meal, provides a reasonable NDS of 90. Milk and dairy products (like pizza cheese and shakes) are rich repositories of riboflavin, as are lean meat, eggs, and enriched bread. The non-fast-food sources include lentils, dried yeast, and liver.

Vitamin B_6 (pyridoxine)

The menus are all low in vitamin B_6. The highest is the pizza meal with an NDS of 58. No analysis is available for the chicken meal, but it is probably low as well. To compensate, try to eat whole-grain products, meats, fish, organ meats,

VITAMIN CONTENT OF FOUR TYPICAL FAST FOOD MEALS

	Calories	Vitamin A (I.U.)	B_1 Thiamin (mg)	B_2 Riboflavin (mg)	B_6 (mg)	B_{12} (ug)	C (mg)	E (mg)	Folacin (ug)	Niacin (mg)	Pantothenic Acid (mg)
MEAL I: SUPER BURGER, REGULAR ORDER OF FRENCH FRIES, VANILLA SHAKE											
Amount	1060	805	.65	.88	.57	3.26	13	2	53	12	2.23
Percent of RDA	55.8	20.1	65	73.3	28.5	108.7	21.7	25	13.3	92.3	40.5
Nutrient Density Score	-	36	116	131	51	195	39	45	24	165	73
MEAL II: FRIED CHICKEN (3 PIECES), ROLL, COLE SLAW, POTATOES											
Amount	990	750	.38	.56	*	*	27	*	*	14	*
Percent of RDA	52.1	18.8	38	46.7	*	*	45	*	*	107.7	*
Nutrient Density Score	-	36	73	90	*	*	86	*	*	207	*
MEAL III: HALF OF 10-INCH CHEESE PIZZA, ICED TEA WITH TWO TEASPOONS OF SUGAR											
Amount	395	598	.24	.41	.24	.92	1	*	*	4	*
Percent of RDA	20.8	15	24	34.2	12.1	30.5	1.7	*	*	30.8	*
Nutrient Density Score	-	72	115	164	58	146	8	*	*	148	*
MEAL IV: FRIED FISH SANDWICH, REGULAR ORDER OF FRENCH FRIES, VANILLA SHAKE											
Amount	990	615	.57	.79	.46	2.18	13	5	45	7	2.47
Percent of RDA	52.1	15.4	57	65.8	23	72.7	21.7	62.5	11.3	53.8	44.9
Nutrient Density Score	-	30	109	126	44	139	42	120	22	103	86

NOTE: This chart contains composite data derived from values provided by fast food chains and standard scientific references. An asterisk substitutes for values that are not available.

The Nutrient Density Score = $\dfrac{\% \text{ RDA for vitamin}}{\% \text{ RDA for calories}} \times 100$.

milk, or wheat germ. Processed or refined foods are lower in B_6 than the raw material. For example, 75 percent of the B_6 is lost in the milling of white flour and is not added back when the flour is enriched.

Vitamin B_{12} (cobalamin)

The menus show excellent levels of B_{12}: The super burger meal scored 195; the pizza, 146, and the fish, 139. No B_{12} analysis is available for the chicken meal, but it contains products of animal origin, which are generally high in B_{12}.

Vitamin C (ascorbic acid)

Vitamin C is quite variable among the menus. The NDS for the pizza meal registers the low of 8 because C is destroyed by the high baking heat. The top score (86) belongs to the chicken. But, in general, fast foods are not notably high in C. However, 4 ounces of orange juice, available at a number of fast food outlets, provide almost 100 percent of the RDA in only 60 calories, boosting the NDS of the pizza meal from eight to 390. A few thick slices of tomato on your burger could also raise your C intake.

Vitamin E (alpha-tocopherol)

Most of the vitamin E in our food supply comes from vegetable fats and oils. That may help explain why the fish meal (deep-fried) scored a satisfying 120, compared to the burger's disappointing NDS of 45. Meat has very little E. To improve your daily intake, rely on wheat germ and whole grains, liver, beans, vegetables, and vegetable oils.

Folacin (folic acid)

Folacin scores—available only for the burger and fish menus—are at critically low levels. The burger scored a measly 24, and the fish 22. Similar scores could be expected of the other two meals because of the absence of green, leafy vegetables. When you eat fast food, make sure your other meals contain green, leafy vegetables (like spinach), cauliflower, broccoli, brussels sprouts, or beets. Whole wheat products and liver are also good sources of folacin. If you are pregnant or taking birth control pills, you should make a special effort to get enough folacin.

Niacin

Niacin is well distributed in all the menus, but the blue ribbon goes to the chicken dinner, which scores a straggering NDS of over 200. If the rest of the day's eating contains enriched cereals, bread, eggs, and lean meats, there should be no difficulty reaching the recommended level of niacin.

MINERALS

Nutritionists divide minerals into two groups, according to how much our bodies need. The first group, the *macro minerals* (calcium, phosphorus, magnesium), is required at levels of 100 mg per day or more. The second group the *trace minerals,* is required in amounts of no more than a few milligrams per day. Fast food lacks good concentrations of some of these nutrients, because soft drinks, shakes, and desserts are loaded with refined sugar, which has no minerals. Also, even though the white flour used for bread products is enriched, the trace minerals (except for iron) are not replaced after processing. Eating whole-grain breads and cereals would help to compensate.

Before you begin gnawing on your pet rock out of concern for your mineral intake, consider how the sample fast food meals rate on the Nutrient Density Score. Again, the chart gives the details for some of the key minerals.

Calcium

Fast food meals tend to be adequate in calcium if you include a shake or milk. (Milk is a better choice for the dieter because it has half the calories for the same amount of calcium). If the fried chicken meal, for example, included milk, the NDS for calcium would soar from 39 to 93. One meal doesn't need any help: the pizza. Because of the cheese, its NDS is 183.

The tortillas used in Mexican food are also high in calcium, because they are pretreated with lime (calcium hydroxide) to improve their cooking properties. Incidentally, the treatment also increases the amount of niacin available from the corn.

Copper

The suggested copper level—there is no firm RDA yet—is 2 to 3 mg per day. None of the meals would go far toward helping you get it. The NDS varies from a high of 38 for the pizza to a low of 16 for the fish. To boost copper intake, eat raisins, lentils, nuts, kidney, and shellfish.

Iodine

A trace mineral, iodine is usually present in generous amounts in fast food because of the use of iodized salt and because iodine compounds are used in maintaining some food preparation machines.

Iron

Fast food, with the exception of Mexican food, seems to be quite low in iron, a trace mineral. The burger meal has an NDS of 49 and the fish meal 27. You really have to try hard to make up the deficiency the rest of the day, because

MINERAL CONTENT OF FOUR TYPICAL FAST FOOD MEALS

	Calories	Calcium (mg)	Copper (mg)	Iodine (ug)	Iron (mg)	Magnesium (mg)	Manganese (mg)	Phosphorus (mg)	Zinc (mg)
MEAL I: SUPER BURGER, REGULAR ORDER OF FRENCH FRIES, VANILLA SHAKE									
Amount	1,060	542	0.29	290	4.9	97	0.51	616	5.2
Percent of RDA	55.8	67.8	11.6	290	27.2	32.3	13.6	77.0	34.7
Nutrient Density Score	-	121	21	520	49	58	24	138	62
MEAL II: FRIED CHICKEN (3 PIECES), ROLL, COLE SLAW, POTATOES									
Amount	990	163	0.44	*	3.1	82	0.61	443	3.9
Percent of RDA	52.1	20.4	17.6	*	17.2	27.3	16.3	55.4	26.0
Nutrient Density Score	-	39	34	*	33	52	31	106	50
MEAL III: HALF OF 10-INCH CHEESE PIZZA, ICED TEA WITH TWO TEASPOONS OF SUGAR									
Amount	395	305	0.20	*	1.1	4.0	0.55	335	2.4
Percent of RDA	20.8	38.1	8.0	*	6.1	13.3	14.7	41.9	16.0
Nutrient Density Score	-	183	38	*	29	64	71	201	77
MEAL IV: FRIED FISH SANDWICH, REGULAR ORDER OF FRENCH FRIES, VANILLA SHAKE									
Amount	990	495	0.21	269	2.5	91	0.47	584	2.2
Percent of RDA	52.1	61.9	8.4	269	13.9	30.3	12.5	73.0	14.7
Nutrient Density Score	-	119	16	516	27	58	24	140	28

NOTE: This chart contains composite data derived from values provided by fast food chains and standard scientific references. An asterisk substitutes for values that are not available.

The Nutrient Density Score = $\frac{\% \text{ RDA for mineral}}{\% \text{ RDA for calories}} \times 100$.

the American diet generally is lacking in iron, particularly for women, who need greater amounts than men. To increase iron intake levels, include in your non-fast-food meals dark green, leafy vegetables, like spinach, as well as nuts, beans, and liver. Another hint: If you drink a glass of orange juice or other citrus fruit product high in vitamin C with your burger, you will increase your body's ability to absorb whatever iron is available in the food.

Magnesium

The fast food menus are below average for magnesium. For example, a fried chicken meal has an NDS of only 52. You can get the missing magnesium from a number of other vegetable and cereal foods, such as 100% bran flakes.

Manganese

Fast food menu items are poor sources of manganese, largely because meat and poultry contain little and fish even less. Although an RDA has not been established for this trace mineral, it is advisable that your diet contain 2.5 to 5 mg per day. The NDS for manganese of the burger and fish meals are both 24. The chicken menu has an NDS of only 31. The pizza meal scores much higher: 71. To increase the manganese in your diet, eat nuts, whole grains, vegetables, and fruits.

Phosphorus

If anything, there is too much phosphorus in fast food, especially because the soft drinks are quite rich in that mineral. When the amount of phosphorus in a person's diet greatly exceeds the amount of calcium, the body's use of calcium may be impaired.

Zinc

The zinc content is highest in the pizza meal (NDS = 77). There is more zinc in the burger meal (NDS = 62) than in the chicken dinner (NDS = 50) or the fish dinner (NDS = 28). Substituting milk for the shake, thereby lowering total calories, improves the zinc picture dramatically. You can add even more zinc to your diet by including in other meals liver, eggs, shellfish (especially oysters), and whole-grain products.

5

THE ADDITIVE DILEMMA

Between bites, a fast food fancier may experience fleeting moments of anxiety about the additives that are probably being ingested along with the meal. Visions of chemicals with terrifying polysyllabic names dance in the eater's head like sugar plum fairies.

It's no fantasy, though. Like other heavily processed foods, the offerings of the chain outlets are laden with a variety of substances that have been added to the raw material for one purpose or another. More than 1,300 additives are approved for use by the federal government, and you can be sure that when you order a large pepperoni and cheese pizza or a hot dog you are getting a hefty share of them. The question is: Should you be worried? The answer is: Maybe.

The first thing to remember is that most additives serve a worthy purpose. They make the food either taste better, look better, last longer, or stay free from germs and spoilage. Some improve physical characteristics like pourability, so that the whole bottle of blue cheese dressing doesn't plop out in two big lumps. In fact, the complicated processing and distribution system that made the fast food industry possible would be impractical without the use of some preservatives and enhancers.

Second, long scary-sounding chemical names don't necessarily mean that a substance is something to be avoided at all costs. You might be tempted to shun a beverage containing jawbreakers like beta-lactalbumin, creatine, lactoglobulin, lactose, ribonucleic acid, and monomagnesium phosphate. But what is it? Nothing more harmful than human mother's milk, widely regarded as the most wholesome food of all.

Many people fear additives because they are not "natural," but naturalness is in the eye of the beholder and is no guarantee of purity or healthfulness. "Vanillin" is a synthetic form of the vanilla flavor so popular in ice cream, but chemically it is exactly the same as the main ingredient in the flavoring extracted from the vanilla bean. In fact, the so-called natural version is not as pure, because it contains residues of oleoresins from the bean. Also, researchers are just beginning to recognize that many so-called natural foods contain naturally occurring toxins, substances that would be poisonous if taken in large doses. Potatoes, for example, contain solanine, a relative of the poison found in the deadly nightshade. It has been estimated that if you eat 120 pounds of french fries or hash browns—which is not untypical of a fast food eater's annual consumption—you take in enough solanine to literally kill a horse if taken all at once.

Even honey, a mainstay of the health food advocates, harbors a potentially carcinogenic substance derived from pollen. But before we launch a movement to ban the beehives, we ought to bear in mind that the toxic or carcinogenic effects of many substances have been demonstrated only in unusually high dosages and sometimes under experimental conditions that are open to varying interpretations. Even when it is agreed that there may be a risk associated with an additive, a reasonable balance may have to be struck between the benefits of using it and the dangers of not using it. Each course has its risks. One of the most controversial additives, the nitrites found in hot dogs and other cured meats, is a suspected carcinogen. However, these nitrites are added to prevent botulism, the often deadly toxic effect of a bacterial contaminant.

Nevertheless, despite all the reasons for using additives, the growing evidence of health hazards does pose a disturbing dilemma for the health-conscious eater, especially one who regularly eats fast food. Since the average person is not a life insurance actuary, it is a bit difficult for us to do a complicated risk-benefit calculation before tearing into a burger. In theory, more accurate and detailed labels, providing a complete roster of the additives in each product, would help the consumer make more intelligent choices, but it might require special skills—perhaps degrees in food technology and biochemistry—even to understand the terms on the label. Besides, there is not much room on a hamburger bun for a label, unless the information could be spelled out in sesame seeds.

There is a growing recognition in the food industry and in the government that it is sound policy at least to reduce the number of food additives and the quantities being used. For example, manufacturers have been experimenting with ways of producing safe meats with no nitrites, or at least much less than had been used in the past.

Ultimately, federal regulatory officials make the decision about which substances are "safe." But we often wonder how diligent the federal regulators are. A familiar television commercial for Hebrew National frankfurters boasts that their kosher products "answer to a higher authority." Most manufacturers, however, content themselves with rendering, as it were, unto Caesar. There is no reviewing body other than the federal government, and, in the eyes of its critics, it is less than impressive in the exercise of its powers.

The enforcement role of the Food and Drug Administration, the main watchdog agency, has been strengthened considerably since the Food, Drug, and Cosmetic Act of 1938 was passed. Under that act, food manufacturers were permitted to use whatever substance they considered safe, and it was up to the FDA to prove additives unsafe. Amendments to the act in 1958 and 1960 shifted the burden of proof to the manufacturers, who since then have had to secure permission from the agency before using a new additive. However, there are two major loopholes in the legislation.

Loophole No. 1: The manufacturers were allowed to continue using substances that had been used as additives for a considerable time without apparent harm. Hundreds of these were included in a category called Generally Recognized as Safe (GRAS), although, critics point out, no scientific studies had ever been done to demonstrate conclusively that these substances did not pose long-term health hazards.

Loophole No. 2: Although the manufacturers are required to prove safety in advance, it is they, or laboratories they commission, who actually conduct the animal testing—not the FDA itself. The critics contend that this arrangement allows the manufacturers, who usually have a large financial stake in the proposed additive, to filter out adverse results or to "interpret" the results in the best light.

The FDA is also subject to a good deal of pressure from manufacturers' lobbies in Washington, either directly or indirectly through friendly members of Congress, although public-interest lobbies have begun to exert countervailing pressures in recent years. Even with the most impartial of approaches, though, it is often difficult to draw from the testing a clear-cut yes or no answer to the question of whether to introduce a new substance or withdraw one already approved.

A key issue is dosage. Almost all chemicals—even water—will produce pathological effects if given in large enough dosages, and scientists often disagree whether tiny amounts of a substance should be banned from human food just because extraordinarily high levels fed to experimental animals produced abnormalities such as tumors or birth defects. Some of the additives are used in such infinitesimal quantities that they are measured in parts-per-billion, amounts that until recently scientists had difficulty even detecting. (To illustrate, one part per billion is the equivalent of a pinch of salt in ten tons of potato chips.)

In one way the FDA's hands are tied, for better or worse. The famous Delaney Clause, part of the 1958 Food Additives Amendment, stipulates that "No additive shall be deemed to be safe if it is found to induce cancer when ingested by man or animals, or if it is found, after tests which are appropriate for the evaluation of the safety of food additives, to induce cancer in man or animals." In effect, the clause sets a rigid limit of "zero tolerance" for any carcinogen, regardless of how small the amounts used or how slight the statistical risk.

The clause has both defenders and detractors. The defenders argue that carcinogens do their lethal work regardless of the amounts involved; there is no threshold beneath which they are ineffective. Moreover, they argue, even if the amount in food poses only a slight risk, it would add to the overall dose of environmental carcinogens to which the average person is exposed, and the cumulative effect might be serious.

The clause caused a storm of controversy when, acting under its authority, the FDA restricted the use of saccharin as a food additive in 1977. The FDA's threat to take saccharin off the market entirely provoked a backlash not only from those who valued saccharin for its claimed benefits in treating obesity and diabetes, but also from the opponents of Big Government, who argued that the FDA should do no more than inform the citizen of the dangers and leave him free to make his own decisions about what to eat. The immediate upshot of the controversy was passage of a Congressional measure that blocked the prohibition until more evidence is available—a poignant demonstration of how attached the public can become to some additives.

What can the individual do until all the facts about additive safety are in? We can assess the dangers for ourselves, given what is known. Here is a quick guide to the major additives likely to be found in fast foods and their associated condiments.

THE ANTI-OXIDANTS

Perhaps the most ominous-sounding additives are a pair of tongue twisters: Butylated hydroxyanisole and butylated hydroxytoluene. To save space on the package labels they are abbreviated as BHA and BHT respectively. The paradox of these twin chemicals is that they are at the same time suspected of (1) posing a health hazard and (2) prolonging life spans.

In general use since the late 1940's, BHA and BHT are commonly employed to prevent rancidity resulting from the breakdown of fats and oils in the presence of oxygen. Added to cooking oils, candy, and prepared foods, they preserve shelf life and freshness, especially in warm weather. But they have come under attack from consumer advocates, who point to experiments which suggest that BHA and BHT might have caused defects ranging from congenital abnormalities to baldness. Follow-up studies by toxicologists, however, found no ill effects even with doses 500 times higher than the average person ingests.

On the contrary, say the champions of the anti-oxidants, BHA and BHT actually have a beneficial effect, because they compensate for what the American diet lacks in vitamin E, a natural anti-oxidant that is thought by some to retard aging. The champions also see another health benefit: They claim that BHA and BHT block the action of other carcinogens and are responsible at least in part for the declining rate of stomach cancer in the United States in recent years.

For now both substances remain government approved. The formula is still BHA + BHT = GRAS. But because of the controversy, a number of manufacturers have begun abandoning them, some turning to the use of vitamin E itself, even though it is not as effective an anti-oxidant as the synthetics.

ARTIFICIAL COLORINGS

Superficial creatures that we are, our appetites are strongly linked to the visual appearance of food. It must not only taste and smell good but also look good. Looking good includes having an attractive color, or at least one that matches our stereotyped notions. Few people would be tempted by a hot dog that looked its natural self, fatty gray, instead of a meaty red that we have come to expect. Manufacturers have been quick to cater to these expectations by routinely adding coloring to our food simply for cosmetic effect. Even fresh food may be gaily painted. For example, coloring is added to some Florida oranges at certain seasons to cover up green spots on the skin.

In the old days, food colorings were extracted from various vegetable products, but because of their higher cost, fluctuating supply, and relative weakness, these extracts were superseded by synthetic dyes derived from coal tar. These blues, greens, yellows, violets, and oranges—often bearing romantic names like Sunset Yellow—are used to brighten up everything from ice cream to breakfast cereals.

In recent years, however, experimental data have implicated several of them in the development of cancer or birth defects in laboratory animals, and some dyes have been taken off the government's approved list. Even the violet dye used by the Agriculture Department for stamping meat carcasses has come under suspicion. Children are a particular cause of concern because they get a heavy dose—as much as 75 mg a day for children aged 6 to 12, the Senate Subcommittee on Nutrition found—largely as a result of drinking so many colorful beverages.

An additional issue has been raised by Dr. Ben Feingold, a San Francisco allergist, who claims that the behavior of hyperactive children can be drastically improved by eliminating from their diets foods containing artificial colors and flavors, and salicylates (a natural component of many fruits, as well as nuts, tomatoes, and cucumbers). Studies so far have failed to support his reports of widespread behavioral improvement. However, a small percentage of hyperactive children do appear to be helped by the additive-free diet. More research is obviously necessary.

The safety of food colorings is undergoing careful scrutiny, and more of them may be "delisted" before long. Of all the additives, these are perhaps the prime targets for abolition because they serve no essential health function and sometimes can be used to disguise poor quality in food. Noodles can be dyed yellow, for example, to simulate higher egg content.

In the meantime you can still feel safe with some food colorings, such as beta-carotene, a yellow coloring often added to margarine. It is actually a nutritional supplement since it converts to vitamin A in the intestines. Some other reliable colorings are xanthophyll (the green in leaves) and the anthocyans (beet color).

ARTIFICIAL FLAVORINGS

Although widely used in place of more expensive natural flavorings, artificial flavorings have been given relatively little scrutiny by the government's safety specialists, because the flavorings are generally used in exceedingly small doses. Most of them, moreover, are merely laboratory copies of the complex combinations of chemicals that give cherries, peaches, strawberries, and so on their natural taste.

Most people's immediate interest in an artificial flavoring is not its possible health effects but its taste. Flavoring is the one additive that the consumer himself can analyze. If you don't like it—if the artificial strawberry flavoring in the ice cream doesn't taste real enough—you are not apt to come back for more.

The flavorings are beginning to come under suspicion, however, because they have not been subjected to as rigorous testing as most other additives, even though many new ones regularly come on the market. (Safrole, the active ingredient in sassafras, was banned in 1960 as a root beer flavoring because it was found to cause liver cancer.) For the time being, though, the regulations leave the consumer in the dark, because the manufacturer need be no more specific than listing the word "artificial flavor" on the package; the chemical names are usually omitted.

CAFFEINE

Caffeine is a stimulant that is found not only in coffee and tea but also in cola drinks. Overconsumption of caffeine can lead to restlessness, irritability, sleeplessness, and nervousness in children as well as adults. A nursing mother also should be aware that the caffeine she drinks will appear in her milk and may affect her infant similarly. Concern has also been expressed about caffeine because in laboratory tests caffeine at high levels proved to be a mutagen (albeit a weak one) causing changes in cells.

You should be conscious of how much caffeine you and your children take in, and it would be prudent to practice moderation. Remember that a young child drinking a can of cola is comparable to an adult drinking four cups of coffee. Here is a list of the caffeine content of beverages commonly served in fast food restaurants.

	mg per serving
Cocoa (5-ounce cup)	9
Coffee, brewed (5-ounce cup)	85
Coffee, freeze-dried (5-ounce cup)	60
Cola (12 ounces)	40 - 70
Iced tea (12-ounce glass)	30
Hot tea (5-ounce cup, steeped 1 minute; increased steeping time increases caffeine content)	50

MOLD AND BACTERIA INHIBITORS

Although bread and cakes are baked at fairly high temperatures, bacteria living at the center of these products may survive the heat treatment, eventually to flourish. Molds may contaminate the loaves later on with carcinogens. For example, the fungus Aspergillus flavus produces aflatoxin, a potent liver carcinogen. Propionates (calcium propionate and sodium propionate) are added to upset the metabolism of the bacteria and molds, keeping them from growing very rapidly.

But although the microorganisms find these chemicals rather unsettling to their routine, the propionates are widely regarded as harmless to people. In fact, they sometimes serve in the body as an energy source, being metabolized into carbon dioxide and water. The propionates also escape suspicion because they occur naturally in some foods. Little more than an ounce of Swiss cheese has enough of these substances to keep several dozen burger buns from getting moldy. Some experts believe that the propionates should be used even more widely than they are, to prevent formation of the potentially carcinogenic molds.

A related microorganism fighter is sodium benzoate. It has been used for generations and is found naturally in many fruits but is effective only under acidic conditions. So its usefulness is restricted to foods like pickles, salad dressing, and carbonated drinks.

The sorbates (calcium, sodium, and potassium sorbate) are newer additions to the anti-mold arsenal. They are effective in both acid and nonacid foods, although they cannot tolerate high temperatures. They also are rather selective weapons: they are more effective against molds than against bacteria. Manufacturers take advantage of that split personality by using sorbates in foods (like cheese) in which it is essential to keep the bacteria alive for flavor while retarding mold growth. Like the propionates, the sorbates are metabolized by the body for energy.

In sum, although no additive is entirely free from suspicion, we know of no ill effects from propionates and sorbates, and they have many beneficial effects.

MONOSODIUM GLUTAMATE (MSG)

Manufacturers of fast food and other processors use large amounts of monosodium glutamate, a derivative of plant protein with the remarkable power of intensifying the flavor of food. This taste-stretcher does its job so well that it can even fool you into believing there is more meat in a dish than there really is.

MSG has been produced and consumed in great quantities since early in this century, when its presence in soy sauce was discovered by a Japanese scientist. But a decade ago a curious symptom called Chinese Restaurant Syndrome (CRS) began appearing in the medical literature, and researchers began to wonder: Did MSG cause CRS?

Characteristic of the syndrome is a burning sensation in the upper chest, neck, or face, accompanied by numbness or a feeling of tigtness; these symptoms appear after eating in a Chinese restaurant. The hypothesis is that the syndrome is a physiological reaction to the liberal dollops of MSG put into the dishes by the Chinese cooks. (MSG is often assumed to be an essential ingredient in Chinese cuisine, but some of the most discriminating chefs disdain its use.)

Estimates of the number of persons experiencing CRS have run as high as 25 percent of the restaurant-eating public. Other researchers consider the true figure to be much lower, perhaps 1 or 2 percent. The syndrome is still under investigation.

MSG has also been implicated in some laboratory studies as a potentially harmful substance. In one study, when it was fed in huge doses to young monkeys, they developed brain lesions. Moreover, its use is opposed by some on the ground that MSG just isn't necessary, and by others on the ground that its sodium content aggravates the general sodium excess in the national diet. In fact, MSG is a rather insidious sodium donor because its taste is only moderately salty, and so you don't notice how much you are absorbing.

Baby food manufacturers have already capitulated, eliminating MSG from the little jars. This was not much of a concession, since it was put there only to make the food taste better when mother dipped her finger in. (Babies apparently do not notice.) Meanwhile, the chemical remains on the GRAS list and will probably stay there until the suspected harmful effects can be proven.

NITRATES AND NITRITES

Nitrates and nitrites might be called the accidental additives. Meat has been cured with salt since ancient times, and much of the salt used in the early days, some of it perhaps scraped off cave walls, contained nitrates and nitrites as impurities. By late Roman times, the ancients had already discovered that these substances had the serendipitous effect of making the meat an attractive red color (by combining with hemoglobin) instead of its natural brown.

Today hot dogs, bacon, and ham owe their appetizing color and characteristic taste largely to the deliberate addition of nitrates and nitrites. These chemicals also serve another purpose: they inhibit the growth of the deadly bacteria known as Clostridium botulinum, the cause of botulism, thereby prolonging refrigerator life. The nitrate-nitrite additives also make the spores of the bacteria heat-sensitive, so that they can be killed when the meat is cooked at reasonable temperatures during processing.

Despite this admirable contribution to public health, the nitrate-nitrite duo has fallen under suspicion because in some circumstances they can combine with substances (secondary amines) to form another group of chemicals, the nitrosamines. These have proven carcinogenic in laboratory animals.

Those who propose eliminating nitrates and nitrites from meat processing have run into powerful opposition. Not only the meat packers but a number of food scientists point out that while the danger to humans from nitrosamines is still theoretical, the risks of deaths from botulism is quite real, particularly since food-handling practices are sometimes inadequate after the meat has left the factory. Also, some researchers have demonstrated that over 80 percent of the nitrates found in a person's saliva are from such natural sources as leafy vegetables. In other words, if the bacon in your bacon-lettuce-tomato sandwich were made nitrate-free, you would still be getting it in the lettuce. Nitrosamines, moreover, have also been discovered in small amounts in beer and scotch, even though nitrates were added to neither.

The government's regulatory policy is to carefully control the maximum levels of nitrates and nitrities that can be added to food. For example, it has banned the addition of nitrates to bacon and lowered the permissible levels of nitrites. With the addition of ascorbates (vitamin C) to bacon, the formation of nitrosamines during cooking is inhibited.

Obviously, it's difficult to determine the nitrate or nitrite level in food you are served in a fast food restaurant, since there is often no label. But con-

sumer-conscious chains may soon, in their menus, sings, or advertising, be high-
lighting dishes that are free of these substances.

SACCHARIN

Saccharin has been used as a sugar substitute for over 70 years, primarily
because it's 350 times sweeter than sugar yet has no calories. But we consume
much more today than we did in the past. More than 44 million adult and teen-
age Americans use the artificial sweetener in some form, most commonly in
soft drinks.

A Great Debate over saccharin erupted in 1977, when it was reported
that huge amounts of the substance fed to laboratory rats caused an increased
incidence of bladder cancer, especially in males. An advisory committee
authorized by Congress confirmed in February 1979 that saccharin was indeed
a carcinogen, although a weak one. To ingest a dose comparable to that of the
rats, a person would have to guzzle over 1,000 cans of diet soda a day. However, a more recent study has found that persons who drank two or more
eight-ounce diet beverages a day had their risk of bladder cancer increased by
60 percent.

Given that saccharin is at least a weak cancer agent, we ought to examine
its claimed benefits carefully. Diabetics and the physicians who treat them say
that it is invaluable. Others argue that even its usefulness to perhaps 6 million
diabetics does not justify its indiscriminate use in food, with or without a
warning label.

What about the seemingly obvious benefits of diet drinks in helping us
stay slim? Surprisingly, there is no scientific evidence to show that saccharin's
use reduces the incidence of obesity. We may just make up for the calories
saccharin saves us by eating other things.

A reasonable solution would be to follow the example of Canada, where
the original rat experiment was performed by making saccharin available as a
self-additive to those who can't do without it (except for the tiny amounts
used to improve the flavor of drugs and toothpaste). In the meantime, one
solution for dieters and other health-conscious eaters is to limit the intake of
saccharin. This is especially important for pregnant women and young children,
since long-term exposure to saccharin is necessary for the harmful effects to
surface.

But don't switch back to sugared soft drinks. That merely aggravates
your overconsumption of refined sugar. Remember that the average 12-ounce
soft drink contains more than eight teaspoons of sugar. A better alternative is
to switch to a drink like iced tea, where a single teaspoon of sugar and only 18
calories does the job. Better yet, drink water.

6

DIETING WITH FAST FOOD

The achievements of the health profession in treating obesity have been compared to those of a football team which has lost every game it ever played. Perhaps the reason is that there have been a rapid succession of coaches, each with a radically different game plan. Barely a month goes by without the appearance of another diet, hailing itself as "revolutionary" and promising instant, effortless weight loss. Sometimes the magic formula is a special combination of foods, a special pill or liquid, or even special clothing. Each new scheme deludes some overweight persons into believing that the basic laws of conservation of energy have been repealed, that they can lose weight without restricting food intake.

These so-called "fad" or "crash" diets claim to take weight off quickly, but they are destined to failure because they are unaccompanied by a fundamental change in eating habits beyond the relatively brief period of active dieting. The dropout rate is high, and lost weight is soon regained. Besides, many diets involve possible health hazards.

Here is a guide to the main diet strategies and their drawbacks.

Low-carbohydrate/high-protein diet

The gimmick of this diet is that you can supposedly lose weight while gorging yourself on unlimited protein, like meat (even with rich sauces), fish, and poultry, so long as you abstain from sugars and starches, like bread, pasta and potatoes. Such diets have been mockingly labeled "thermodynamic miracles," because food energy is supposed to dissipate miraculously instead of being turned into body weight.

On a low-carbohydrate diet initial weight loss is rapid but is mostly water, and once even a small amount of carbohydrates are reintroduced into the diet, the water weight is quickly regained. Among the dangers are extreme

39

fatigue, fainting, calcium depletion, aggravation of undiagnosed kidney diseases, and increased uric acid levels, precipitating a gout attack. Also, the diet increases the intake of cholesterol and fat, including saturated fat.

High-carbohydrate/low-protein/low-fat diet

Again, there is supposedly no need to count calories, but this time the gimmick is reversed. You stay away from meat, poultry, seafood, milk, and dairy products but indulge in starchy foods. The main objection is the same: If your calorie total is high, regardless of the source, you will not lose weight.

You may eat fewer calories on this diet because starchy foods are so bulky. But since Americans are accustomed to eating much meat, it is difficult to stay on such a diet.

Some exponents of high-carbohydrate diets have claimed that you can aim the diet like a laser, reducing weight on a specific part of your body. The evidence, however, indicates that if you have abnormally large fat deposits, they will still be disproportionately large even if your overall weight drops.

Starvation diet

This diet has the virtue of simplicity. You avoid all food, drink nothing but water, and lose a pound a day. However, the long-term results are discouraging. Once the ephemeral burst of will power is over, the weight is usually regained. Besides, the dangers are legion. They include dehydration, nausea, dizziness, fatigue, high uric acid levels (which can precipitate gout attacks), and depletion of minerals such as potassium, calcium, and magnesium. Kidney and liver functions can also be affected. Starvation diets should never be attempted without close medical supervision.

Protein-sparing fast

This is a variant of the starvation diet. In some versions the dieter ingests a small amount of "predigested" liquid protein of poor quality to compensate for a major disadvantage of fasting—the body's tendency to cannibalize itself by burning vital muscles and organ tissue (the "lean body mass") for fuel. Weight loss tends to be quick but short-lived once the dieter goes back to regular food. The hazards include those of low-carbohydrate diets, as well as cardiac arrhythmia, probably caused by potassium depletion. The Food and Drug Administration has identified such diets as a contributing factor in a number of deaths and has considered requiring warning labels on the liquid protein packages. This diet should be attempted only under careful medical supervision, and only using the high-quality protein found in lean meat, fish, and poultry.

Vegetarian diet

In principle, there is nothing wrong with a vegetarian weight-reducing diet. There are even some important advantages: it tends to be high in fiber and low in cholesterol, especially if the dieter also avoids eggs, as many vegetarians do. However, if you do not eat eggs, cheese, or milk, it is crucial to choose vegetables foods with high-quality protein, such as soybeans, and to mix foods in such a way that their proteins are complementary. Beans and rice are one such combination. Many people find it difficult to put so much effort into deciding what to eat. Also, strict vegetarians may have to take vitamin B_{12} supplements.

Macrobiotic diet

This group of diets relies mainly on whole-grain cereal, fish, and selected vegetables. The most drastic of them calls for 100 percent brown rice. Few people can stay on such spartan regimens for long, and that is fortunate. Although their proponents claim the diets can cure everything from air sickness to varicose veins, eating only brown rice will soon lead to depletion of nutrients, including protein, calcium, and vitamins A and C. Scurvy is one likely outcome.

Special food diet

A number of diets center around eating specific foods or supplements, like bananas and milk, lecithin and kelp, and even ice cream. The diets are acceptable to those who happen to like the favored food—kelp is not everyone's idea of lunch—but there is a tendency to become bored and lose interest in the restricted menu. Besides, there still is no magic weight disappearance unless eating the special dish helps you in some way to reduce your overall caloric intake. Consuming 5,000 calories worth of bananas each day is likely to make you simply a fat banana eater.

BEYOND THE BLITZ

Unlike the foregoing regimens, *The Fast Food Diet* can have long-lasting effects because it is intended for more than just a brief "blitz." Its aim is to permanently adjust eating habits. That is a realistic goal, because the diet takes into account people's preferences for fast food. In other words, it rolls with the punches. It also emphasizes *balance* in the diet, so that the dieter is assured of getting all the nutrients needed, even though the fast foods themselves may be lacking in some respects.

Before you attempt to diet, you should make sure that you really need to lose weight, In the laboratory, there are a variety of technical methods for determining the proportion of fat in a person's body; this is the most accurate indicator. These methods include such arcane procedures as weighing a person underwater, measuring potassium isotopes in the body with a radiation counter, and X-raying the soft tissue. Outside the laboratory these tests are obviously impractical, but you can judge fairly well whether you are over-weight by using any one of seven simple self-assessment techniques:

1. *The Belly-Button Test.* With a tape measure, measure the circum-ference of your waist at the navel. Then measure your chest circumference at the nipples. If the navel measurement is larger than the chest measurement, you have too much fat in the abdomen. This condition is commonly known as Rubber Tire Syndrome.

2. *The 36-Inch Test.* Subtract your waist measurement in inches from your height in inches. If the result is less than 36, you are overweight.

3. *The Five-Foot Test.* The ideal weight for a person exactly five feet (60 inches) tall is 100 pounds for women and 106 pounds for men. If you are taller than five feet, add five pounds (women) or six pounds (men) for each inch above 60. That is *your* ideal weight. If you are more than 20 percent heavier than the ideal, you are overweight.

4. *The Ruler Test.* Lie flat on your back and place a ruler longitudinally (in the head-to-toe-direction) on your stomach. If the ruler does not touch both the pubis and the bottom of the rib cage at the same time, but rather tilts toward one or the other, you are overweight.

5. *The Pinch Test.* Pinch the skin and underlying fat at several points on your body: the backs of the upper arms, the side of the lower chest, and the back just below the shoulder blade. If there is more than an inch between your thumb and forefinger, you are probably overweight. (This test is more useful for people under 50, because more than half their fat is found just under the skin.)

6. *The Longevity Test.* Another possibility is to measure yourself against the standard table of desirable adult (25 years and up) weights com-piled by the Metropolitan Life Insurance Company. The table is shown here in modified form. For those between 18 and 25, subtract one pound for each year under 25. These weights are rather generous, so you can be sure that if you weigh 20 percent more than the average for your weight, you are over-weight.

7. *The Who's-the-Fairest-of-Them-All Test.* View yourself nude in a full-length mirror. Ask yourself, honestly, whether you look overweight.

Once you have decided that you are overweight and have determined how many pounds you need to lose, the next step is to determine how fast the excess should come off. (Incidentally, it's always a good idea to check with your doctor before dieting.) The basic inescapable axiom of weight reduction

RECOMMENDED WEIGHT IN RELATION TO HEIGHT*

Height		Men		Women	
Feet	Inches	Average	Range	Average	Range
4	10	-	-	102	92-119
4	11	-	-	104	94-122
5	0	-	-	107	96-125
5	1	-	-	110	99-128
5	2	123	112-141	113	102-131
5	3	127	115-144	116	105-134
5	4	130	118-148	120	108-138
5	5	133	121-152	123	111-142
5	6	136	124-156	128	114-146
5	7	140	128-161	132	118-150
5	8	145	132-166	136	122-154
5	9	149	136-170	140	126-158
5	10	153	140-174	144	130-163
5	11	158	144-179	148	134-168
6	0	162	148-184	152	138-173
6	1	166	152-189	-	-
6	2	171	156-194	-	-
6	3	176	160-199	-	-
6	4	181	164-204	-	-

*Height without shoes, weight without clothes. Adapted from the Table of the Metropolitan Life Insurance Co. Source: Fogarty International Center Conference on Obesity.

is the Calorie Deficit Principle. Simply put, to lose one pound of fat during any given period of time, most people need to eat 3,500 calories less than they burn up as energy in that time. If you manage to achieve such a deficit over the course of a week, you will lose a pound in that week. (If you have a surplus of 3,500 calories in that week, however, you will gain a pound.)

A person who takes in exactly as many calories as she burns up will remain at energy equilibrium and maintain her weight. A chart in Chapter 3 gave the calories necessary for maintenance. These vary according to the following factors.

1. *Your weight:* The more you weigh, the more calories it takes to fuel the body mass. The difference between maintenance levels may be quite small. At age 35, for example, the difference between a woman maintaining her weight at 128 pounds and 143 pounds is only 200 calories a day.
2. *Your age:* The older you are, the fewer calories it takes to maintain weight. If you keep on eating the same amount as you age, you will find obesity creeping up on you.

3. *Activity:* The more physically active you are, the more calories it
takes to maintain weight.

The Fast Food Diet provides 1,200 calories for the day, a level that should
result in a sufficient calorie deficit in most persons to allow them to lose up
to three pounds per week. That is a safe and reasonable rate of loss. No one
should diet on fewer than 1,000 calories for an extended period. It is a hard
regimen to maintain, and it could prove unhealthy because of the difficulty
in achieving nutritional balance. *The Fast Food Diet* assumes light physical
activity; by doing more strenuous activity, you can lose even more.

BREAKING THE OVERWEIGHT HABIT

In general, the best way to look at your overweight problem is as an overall
pattern of eating and exercise habits. Because you are overweight, by definition those habits are inappropriate. The only lasting solution is to change the
habits, to replace them with newer and more healthful ones. Total change, of
course, is hard to take, and that is one reason why the so-called revolutionary
cure-alls fail. It's far better to let yourself carry on with some of the old ways
while seeking to abandon others. In this diet, we assume that one of the habits
to which you are particularly attached is eating fast food, so we will build in
that preference while working to change some of the surrounding habits that
add up to obesity.

To make significant changes in your eating patterns, it is essential that all
behaviors relating to food intake be carefully recorded and analyzed. Here are
the three basic phases of self-analysis:

Phase I. Record-Keeping

Keep accurate records. The purpose of record-keeping is to make you aware of
what and how much you eat. Often, the awareness that record-keeping brings
will in itself help you cut back on total food intake. Entries must be made
immediately, so you must always have the record with you. Carry a little
notebook. Make sure the entries are detailed and, above all, honest. You are
most likely to cheat on them when overeating and that is precisely the behavior
that needs to be most accurately recorded.

This is what to write in your record book:

Time. List the time that each meal begins and the time it ends. Every
discrete episode of eating must be considered a "meal." Every time
you take some food, even pop a gumdrop in your mouth, it's a meal.
Type and amount of food. List the kind of food and your best estimate
of the size of the portion. Use either the weight or the number of

pieces. (For example, three pieces of fried fish, 4 ounces of cola, half a pound of peanuts.) Also list the calories.

Hunger level. Judge how hungry you are just before you sit down to eat, on a scale of 0 to 5. If you are not hungry at all, it is 0; if you are as hungry as you have ever been, it is 5.

Place. This is the scene-of-the-crime report. Where did you eat the food? If at home, was it in the kitchen, dining room, bedroom, or attic? If you ate away from home, enter the name of the restaurant and whether the meal was at a counter or a table. Don't forget to record any eating that may occur while walking, driving your car, or riding in a bus or taxi.

Physical position. When you ate, were you standing, sitting, lying down, or in some other position?

Related activity. What were you doing while you were eating? Were you reading, watching television, talking on the telephone? Note whether you are alone or with others.

Mood. Just before you ate, were you feeling tense, depressed, elated, bored?

Here is a sample record-keeping form:

Date _____

Time		Type and Amount of Food	Calories	Hunger Level 0-5	Place Eaten	Physical Position When Eating	Related Activity	Mood
Start	Finish							

This may look like a lot of effort, and it is. But strict record-keeping is worthwhile, if only because you may decide not to have a snack just to save yourself the trouble of filling out the form.

Phase II. Analyzing the Records

Keep the records for one week before starting your diet. Then look over your notes and ask yourself these questions:

How many meals in all did I have during the week? (Remember, a meal is defined as any discrete period of eating.)

How many meals took 0 to 4 minutes, 5 to 10 minutes, 11 to 20 minutes, more than 20 minutes?

How many times did I eat in the dining room, living room, bedroom? In my car, on the bus or train? While walking, in the office, in a restaurant?

How many times during the week did I eat while standing, sitting, lying down?

How many meals did I eat alone? How many when I was with others?

How many meals did I eat without doing anything else? How many while reading or watching television?

How many meals did I eat while my hunger rating was 0 to 2? How many 3 to 5?

How many meals did I eat while I was neutral? Tense? Depressed?

Phase III. Making Changes

The answers to these questions profile your daily eating routine. Starting from this profile, you can make adjustments. In the first place, if your food records show that you ate more than 30 meals during the week according to the strict definition of "meal," make a conscious effort to eat less frequently during the coming week. High-frequency eating tends to increase food consumption. When you have to think about whether you are exceeding your meal quota, you will skip opportunities to slip some food into your mouth.

Calculate your calorie total for the week. If it's higher than necessary to maintain the weight that you *should* be at, start setting calorie limits. Gradually lower the limits.

If you eat in many places, you can gain control of unplanned food consumption by picking one spot in your home for meals and sticking to it. Designating only one place for eating will make it more difficult to absorb calories casually. Being free to munch at will in every corner of the house offers too many opportunities to wander off and curl up with a ham sandwich.

If your pattern is to eat while doing something else, such as reading, watching television, or driving a car, make sure that from now on your meals are unaccompanied by diversionary activities. Heightened awareness of your meals will prevent Overeater's Amnesia, which makes you conveniently forget how much you've taken in that day.

Also try slowing your pace. Most overweight persons rush down their food. Prolong meals so they last more than 20 minutes each. Put down your fork or spoon after each bite. Chew leisurely and swallow slowly. Halfway through your meal, stop eating and relax for two minutes. This is especially important while you are eating fast food, which tends to go down with lightning speed.

If you eat large meals, use a smaller plate, and leave some food on it when you finish. This is almost impossible for some people, but you can nominate your least favorite food as the leftover. It may help not to tell your friends and family that you are dieting. Some people take a perverse delight in trying to get you to break your diet "just this once."

Don't let yourself eat just because of the mood you happen to be in. If you tend to fill your mouth whenever you are bored or depressed, you are using food as a psychological crutch and are gaining excess calories unnecessarily. Eat only when you are truly hungry. It is surprising how many people don't know what hunger is because they never let themselves go without food long enough to experience the sensation.

The overall goal is to *plan* your eating rather than letting it happen randomly. This is especially true when you are dealing with high-temptation items like fast food. Following are some hints on how to deal with your impulses:

1. Decide at which restaurant you will eat, and set a ceiling on the number of calories you will have. Use the charts at the back of this book to organize your menu.
2. Make your visit to the restaurant coincide with a main meal time, so that it serves as lunch or supper rather than as a snack.
3. Don't order dessert before you've finished the main part of the meal. Once you've eaten some food, you may feel satisfied enough to do without dessert.
4. If you are tempted by ice cream or dessert, plan to eat it at a time when you are relatively full. That will help you savor the pleasure, so that the craving is satisfied. Eat small amounts.
5. Plan the rest of the day's eating so that you do not exceed a fixed calorie total and so that you get a balanced diet.

ACHIEVING BALANCE

The daily and weekly meal plans in this book are examples of how to build fast food into a well-rounded but calorically modest diet. The key to meeting known and still unknown nutritional need is to eat a variety of foods, choosing some from each of the food groups. They are as follows:

The Vegetable and Fruit Group

Have four or more servings a day. A serving equals one orange, one small banana, a half cup of vegetables, or one medium potato.

Variety within the group is also important. Not all fruits and vegetables provide the same nutrients, although most foods in this group provide vitamins A and C as well as fiber. Make sure to have one serving of citrus fruit so you get enough vitamin C. Dark green vegetables contribute vitamin A, riboflavin, folacin, iron, and magnesium. Nearly all fruits and vegetables are low in fat, and none contains cholesterol.

The Bread and Cereal Group

Have four or more servings a day. One serving is one slice of whole-grain or enriched bread, one ounce of ready-to-eat cereal, or ½ to ¾ cup cooked cereal. Other foods in this group are biscuits, muffins, waffles, pancakes, pasta, grits, cornmeal, rice, barley, and bulgar wheat.

Whole grains are usually a good source of folacin and other B vitamins, iron, magnesium, and fiber. Most ready-to-eat breakfast cereals are selectively fortified at higher levels than natural grain products and may have additional nutrients such as vitamins A, B_{12}, C, and D. But you get better variety from whole-grain cereals. If you prefer a ready-to-eat cereal, choose one with a minimum of sugar and don't add extra. Minimize intake of highly refined foods.

The Milk and Milk Products Group

Have two servings per day. One serving is one cup of milk, one ounce of cheese, one cup of plain yogurt, 1½ cups of ice cream, or two cups of cottage cheese. Foods in this group are a good source of calcium, vitamin A (skim milk products are fortified with A), B_2, B_6, and B_{12}, and some are fortified with vitamin D.

The Protein Group

Have two or more servings. One serving is 2 to 3 ounces of lean, cooked meat, poultry, or fish. The following are equivalent to one ounce of meat: one egg; ½ to ¾ cup of cooked dry beans, dry peas, soybeans, or lentils; two tablespoons of peanut butter; or ¼ to ½ cup of nuts, sesame seeds, or sunflower seeds.

In addition to high-quality protein, this group provides phosphorus and vitamins B_6 and B_{12} (animal products only). Various foods in this group also provide additional nutrients, such as zinc (from red meats and oysters), vitamin A (liver and egg yolks), and magnesium (dry beans, peas, soybeans, and nuts). Polyunsaturated fatty acids and the essential fatty acids are provided by the seeds.

The Fats, Sweets, and Alcohol Group

For those persons who are restricting their calories, servings from this group should be minimal. Eaters of fast food typically consume more than is advisable of fats and sweets.

In general, if you choose a good variety of food, you will get all the vitamins and minerals you need. But you may want to take supplements if you fall into any of the following categories:

1. If you eliminate any of the food groups or fixate on one or two of them.

2. If you are dieting and your calorie intake is less than 1,200 calories per day.

3. If you are pregnant. It may be difficult for you to get enough iron and folacin. Be sure to check with your physician for guidelines as to when and how much of a supplement to take.

4. If you smoke. You may need extra vitamin C.

5. If you drink heavily. Alcohol affects the absorption and utilization of some nutrients: some of the B vitamins (B_1, B_6, and folacin) and minerals (magnesium, zinc, potassium).

6. If you are 65 years or older. As you get older, the absorption and utilization of certain nutrients may decrease.

7. If you suffer from a medical condition requiring supplementation. Check with your physician. Also, some prescription drugs interfere with nutrient utilization and necessitate supplementation. For example, if you are taking birth control pills, folacin and B_6 levels tend to be low.

It is important not only to choose your food well but to cook it properly. Here are some cooking tips for dieters:

1. Cook and serve vegetables without butter or margarine. Each pat of fat adds at least 50 calories.

2. Steam or cook vegetables quickly in only a little water. Vitamins like folacin are water soluble, and others are destroyed by prolonged cooking.

3. Use vinegar, fresh lemon juice, or even tomato juice (less than 5 calories per tablespoon) in place of salad dressing (60 to 100 calories per table-spoon). Another alternative is low-calorie dressing (15 to 40 calories per tablespoon).

4. Grill or broil meats rather than frying them. Each tablespoon of oil adds 120 calories.

5. Pay attention to portion size. Most people underestimate the size and caloric content of meats and overestimate the caloric content of starchy foods. Weigh all meat and cheese until you become expert in judging. (Note: A postage scale is cheaper than a kitchen scale and more accurate for weighing ounces).

6. Trim off all visible fat. An average T-bone steak has about 100 calories per ounce; if well trimmed, it has 46 calories per ounce.

7. To minimize vitamin loss, use *fresh* fruits and vegetables where possible, and don't store for long periods of time.

THE EXERCISE FACTOR

Besides food intake, activity remains the one big factor that is very much in your control. If you kept your food intake at the same level, you might be able to achieve a calorie deficit just by upping the activity level. Even better is to decrease food intake as well as increasing activity, because it takes a good deal more effort than you might think to dissipate the energy in some of our favorite meals. Some examples of the amount of activity required are shown in the chart on the following page.

As the chart suggests, isolated bursts of activity won't make the pounds vanish. But it does make sense to raise your overall level of activity, because the sedentary lifestyle is thought by most researchers to be closely linked to the national penchant for paunchiness.

The connection between inactivity and obesity seems to be especially strong in women. Several studies have demonstrated the point. In one, overweight women were found to have walked half as many miles (14.4) in a week as normal weight women; in another, overweight girls at summer camp were found to spend the same amount of time in the pool as normal girls, but they swam less and floated more. The lazy life apparently starts early: Some obese toddlers have been shown to eat no more than others but to spend less time toddling.

You're mistaken if you think that if you exercise you will start eating like a lumberjack. In fact, exercise may pack a double whammy by reducing your appetite as well as burning calories. Studies of formerly sedentary laboratory animals showed that exercise decreased their desire for food.

Persons over 35 should check with a physician before starting vigorous exercise, but even less-than-robust activity helps.

Walking at least 30 minutes each day has been shown to be highly effective in helping people lose an average of 20 pounds over the course of a year. For that reason, the dieter should have two measuring instruments, a scale and a pedometer. A pedometer is the clocklike instrument that hikers use to record how far they've walked. It is inexpensive and can be purchased at most sporting goods stores. Wear the pedometer for a week, at the end of each day recording the number of miles walked. Once you have found the daily average, gradually increase it, setting new goals for yourself each week. As the miles go up, weight will come down.

Increasing your walking will take some ingenuity at first. Stride around the house during television commercials. Get off the bus ten blocks early on your way to and from work and walk the rest of the way (annual weight loss: 3 pounds). Ride the elevator only part way up twice a day, taking the stairs at least three floors (annual weight loss: up to 10 pounds).

ACTIVITY

Food	Total Calories	Watching TV on the Couch	Walking the Dog (2 mph)	Swimming 20 yards/minute	Calisthenics	Moderate Tennis	Downhill Skiing	Jogging (4.5 mph)
1 Munchkin (yeast-raised) **Dunkin' Donuts**	26	20	8	5	4	4	3	3
1 breaded fried shrimp **Arthur Treacher's**	54	42	16	11	8	8	6	6
1 small Orange Julius **Orange Julius**	149	115	45	31	22	21	17	16
Vanilla shake **Jack in the Box**	342	263	104	71	51	49	38	36
Big Mac **McDonald's**	541	416	164	113	80	78	61	58
Rib-eye steak platter **Rustler Steak House**	802	617	243	167	119	116	90	85
Triple hamburger with cheese **Wendy's**	1,036	797	314	216	153	149	116	110

*Calculated for a person weighing 150 pounds.

You might even walk to the fast food restaurant instead of driving thereby helping to burn up the calories in the process of getting them. (If i makes you feel better, you can still order from the drive-through window. Some restaurants encourage physical activity by having a bike-up window fo cyclists. At the very least, park your car in the spot furthest from the restau rant.

7

THE DIETER'S GUIDE TO FAST FOOD CHAINS

Fast food fanciers usually know what and where they like to eat, but they are less clear about the nutritional content of their meals. In this section, the menus of leading fast food chains and popular family-style restaurants are analyzed so that you can make more informed choices.

Each entry discusses the chain's offerings and suggests diet strategies for eating there. A chart shows the number of calories in each menu item and the proportion of the calories contributed by protein, fat, and carbohydrate. (For an explanation of Nutrient Density Scores used in this chapter, see Chapter 4.)

In addition, this guide provides daily diet plans that incorporate one meal from each chain. The meals for the rest of the day balance food intake according to sound nutritional principles. At the end of the chapter is a calorie analysis of the most common condiments, drinks, and salad bar ingredients.

The charts are based mainly upon data provided by the chains. In some instances, the nutritional values have been calculated by the authors, using United States Department of Agriculture tables and food weights reported by the chains. The charts should be viewed only as a general guide to meal planning. For the most part, the data is derived from analyses of samples of food served, and significant variations may occur. Also, menu items may vary according to the availability of ingredients and may be reformulated periodically.

ARBY'S

Although Arby's ten-plus gallon cowboy hat symbol is reminiscent of the old West, the chain's origins are purely Ivy League. Two brothers, one a graduate of Cornell University's School of Hotel Administration and the other from the University of Pennsylvania's equally prestigious Wharton School of Finance, decided to use their expensive education to champion the inexpensive roast beef sandwich.

Arby's, which stands for the initials "R.B." of the Raffel Brothers (not for roast beef), provides an alternative to the more traditional fast food fare. Its menu concentrates on sandwiches—various combinations of roast beef, cheese, ham, and turkey, topped with mayonnaise-based dressing, lettuce, and tomatoes.

Roast beef is the house special. Arby's describes its meat as follows: "A self-basting beef roast made to our strict specifications with trimmed boneless beef chunks, combined with just enough chopped beef for 9-12 percent fat." However, the roast beef sandwich provides 38.5 percent of its *calories* in the form of fat. (The club sandwich is the highest fat item—48 percent of calories—mainly because of the dressing.)

Those watching their salt intake should also be aware that the roast beef sandwich comes with 880 mg of sodium. The Super roast beef sandwich contains 1,420 mg—almost half the R.D.A.

The Junior roast beef sandwich is a bonus for dieters at 220 calories. The Super roast beef contains twice the amount of beef (3 ounces) but nearly three times the calories (620), mainly because of the dressing and the larger roll. The Super's lettuce and tomato account for only 15 extra calories.

At hand at every table are squeeze bottles of Arby's own brands of barbecue sauce and Horsey (mild horseradish) Sauce. Using them to perk up the roast beef sandwich adds fewer calories than a heavy topping, and if you like souvenirs you can buy a bottle to take home. You can also save calories by putting cole slaw on the roast beef sandwich instead of the topping.

Here's a sample day built around lunch at Arby's:

	Calories
BREAKFAST:	
1 sliced, small banana with	85
1 cup Wheat Chex cereal and	165
3/4 cup skim milk	66
Coffee or tea	0
	316
LUNCH AT ARBY'S:	
Arby's Junior roast beef sandwich	220
(Try to pay extra for 2 tomato slices and lettuce.)	(10)
Cole slaw	83
Coffee, tea, or iced tea	0
	303(313)
DINNER:	
3/4 cup tomato juice	35
Sauteed chicken livers:	245
5 oz. chicken livers	
10 sliced, small mushrooms (fresh)	

	Calories
1/2 sliced onion	
1 tablespoon margarine	
Cook in a no-stick frying pan and serve on	
1 slice whole wheat toast	65
1 cup broccoli	40
1 large wedge lettuce (2 cups) with	16
2 tablespoons low-calorie salad dressing	30
1 two-inch slice honeydew melon with lemon juice	49
Coffee or tea	0
	480

SNACK:

1 cup skim milk	88

TOTAL CALORIES FOR DAY = 1,187 (1,197)

ARBY'S®

Item	Calories	Protein grams	Protein % calories	Fat grams	Fat % calories	Carbohydrate grams	Carbohydrate % calories
Sandwich							
Roast beef	350	22	25.1	15	38.5	32	36.4
Beef 'n' Cheese	450	27	24.0	22	44.0	36	32.0
Super roast beef	620	30	19.5	28	40.9	61	39.6
Junior roast beef	220	12	22.6	9	38.0	21	39.4
Swiss King	660	34	20.6	34	46.2	55	33.2
Ham 'n Cheese	380	23	24.4	17	40.6	33	35.0
Turkey	410	24	23.4	19	41.6	36	35.0
Turkey Deluxe	510	28	21.9	24	42.2	46	35.9
Club	560	30	21.4	30	48.0	43	30.6
Cole slaw* (3 oz.)	83	1	4.5	7	68.3	6	27.0
French fries* (2.5 oz)	211	3	5.6	11	46.0	26	48.4
Apple Turnover* (3 oz.)	300	2	2.9	19	55.8	31	41.3

*Calculated on the basis of weight provided by Arby's.

ARTHUR TREACHER'S FISH & CHIPS

When Arthur Treacher's appeared on the American scene, fast food fans all over the country wondered: Who is Arthur Treacher? And what is a chip? Those who had seen the English film actor's portrayal of the perfect butler knew the answer to the first question. As to the second, the story of the chip reflects the great cultural gulf separating British civilization from that of the rest of Europe. The continental french fry is thin, delicate, rather like a shoe-string potato. The British chip, on the other hand, is robust and meaty, and can stay crisp even if it rains all day.

American eaters generally have accepted British-style potato eating. Many balk, however, at going totally native by dousing their fried fish with vinegar. The tables at Arthur Treacher's are stocked with pungent, mahogany-brown malt vinegar, but the bottles often stay full. The more familiar ketchup dispensers seem to get heavier use. So much for the union of the English-speaking peoples.

Although the chain made its name purveying seafood, other imaginative uses for the deep-fry batter have been found, such as wrapping it around a hot dog. Mounted on a stick, like a deep-fried lollypop, the Krunch Pup has its devotees, but dieters should be aware that the batter adds about 80 calories to the hot dog's already generous endowment, bringing the total to 203. And the Krunch Pup gets 65 percent of its calories from fat.

The highlight meal is the seafood platter, an assortment of fried fish, shrimp, clams, and oysters, set off by a pair of hush puppies (onion-flavored corn meal fritters) and cole slaw. It's tempting, but the total calorie count, almost 1,100, would devastate most diets. The fish sandwich (440) is a more modest alternative, especially if you do without the generous layer of tartar sauce under the top half of the bun; that accounts for almost 150 calories.

A satisfying dinner also can be put together as shown below. You can use the lemon supplied in packets to ease the loss of tartar sauce. The breakfast and lunch menus also help compensate somewhat for the dinner's fat content (45 percent of calories) and relatively low levels of vitamin A, B vitamins, calcium, magnesium, iron, zinc, and copper. Using the salad bar available at some Arthur Treacher's outlets may also help provide these nutrients.

	Calories
BREAKFAST:	
1/6 of 5-inch cantaloupe	20
1 cup 100% Bran Flakes with	150
1 tablespoon raisins and	29
3/4 cup skim milk	66
Tea or coffee	0
	265

	Calories

LUNCH:

Spinach salad:	215
3 1/2 ounces fresh spinach	
1 quartered hard-boiled egg	
1 medium tomato, cut in wedges	
4 sliced large mushrooms (fresh)	
2 tablespoons cooked chick peas	
Thinly sliced Bermuda onion	
Garlic wine vinegar or lemon wedges	
1 slice whole wheat bread	65
1 cup skim milk	88
	368

DINNER AT ARTHUR TREACHER'S:

Chowder	112
1 piece fried fish	178
Chips	276
Coffee or tea	0
	566

TOTAL CALORIES FOR DAY = 1,199

ARTHUR TREACHER'S FISH & CHIPS

Item	Calories	Protein		Fat		Carbohydrate	
		grams	% calories	grams	% calories	grams	% calories
Chowder	112	4.6	16.4	5.4	43.5	11.2	40.1
Fish (2 pieces)	355	19.2	21.5	19.8	50.0	25.4	28.5
Chicken (2 pieces)	369	27.1	29.4	21.6	52.7	16.5	17.9
Shrimp (7 pieces)	381	13.1	13.8	24.2	57.5	27.2	28.7
Krunch Pup	203	5.4	10.6	14.8	65.7	12.0	23.7
Fish sandwich	440	16.4	14.9	24.0	49.2	39.4	35.9
Chicken sandwich	413	16.2	15.7	19.2	41.8	44.0	42.5
Chips	276	4.0	5.8	13.2	43.3	34.9	50.9
Cole slaw	123	1.0	3.3	8.2	60.4	11.1	36.3
Lemon Luv	276	2.6	3.8	13.9	45.3	35.1	50.9

BASKIN-ROBBINS ICE CREAM

The ancient art of ice cream making was apparently another first for Chinese inventiveness, but unfortunately for Occidental dieters the secret was given away. However it made its way to America, ice cream has been developed into an array of 450 flavors by another inventive outfit, Baskin-Robbins, the California-based chain. The 31 flavors that are in each store each month (they are rotated) sorely tempt the calorie-restricted.

Luckily, there are some ways to include some icy treats in your daily fare. For under 100 calories you can indulge in a chilled fruit salad yogurt or, for even fewer, treat yourself to the elegantly titled daiquiri ice (84 calories). Generally, the yogurts and sherbets have less fat than the ice creams (13 percent versus 50 percent) but more sugar.

If you want an ice cream, remember that some flavors are lower in calories than others. Strawberry has 141 per scoop, compared to 181 for French vanilla. Also, skip the sugar cone (abut 40 calories) unless you're one of those who thinks it's the best part. Concentrate on eating the ice cream slowly, stretching out the pleasure as long as possible. Eating quickly will just make you pine for another. While you're eating, you can think about all the calcium you are getting. The Nutrient Density Score for calcium in a scoop of vanilla is 137.

Here is a full day with a Baskin-Robbins dessert and a snack built in:

	Calories
BREAKFAST:	
3/4 cup tomato juice	35
3/4 cup Wheatena cereal with	115
1 tablespoon raisins and	29
3/4 cup skim milk	66
Coffee or tea	0
	245
LUNCH:	
Tuna fish salad:	165
3 1/2 ounces tuna fish (water packed) on	
lettuce leaf	
1 sliced medium tomato	
1 sliced medium cucumber (unpeeled)	
3 radishes	
1 slice whole wheat bread	65
1 large tangerine	46
Coffee or tea	0
	276

	Calories

DINNER WITH BASKIN-ROBBINS DESSERT:

Hungarian chicken:	220
1 small chicken breast barbecued or broiled with lemon juice and paprika	
1 cup zucchini	22
3 sliced radishes and 1 cup watercress with 2 tablespoons low-calorie salad dressing	40
1 slice whole wheat bread	65
1/2 teaspoon margarine	17
Coffee or tea	0
1 scoop Baskin-Robbins chocolate ice cream	165
	529

SNACK:

Strawberry treat:	142
Mix in a blender or food processor	
1 cup skim milk	
1 cup frozen strawberries (unsweetened)	

TOTAL CALORIES FOR DAY = 1,192

BASKIN-ROBBINS ICE CREAM

Item	Calories	Protein		Fat		Carbohydrate	
		grams	% calories	grams	% calories	grams	% calories
(servings = one scoop)							
Vanilla	147	2.6	7.1	8.2	50.3	15.6	42.6
Chocolate	165	2.8	6.8	7.9	43.4	20.4	49.8
Strawberry	141	2.5	7.1	7.7	48.9	15.6	44.0
French vanilla	181	2.9	6.3	11.8	58.7	15.9	35.0
Chocolate fudge	178	2.7	6.2	9.1	46.0	21.3	47.8
Pralines 'n' cream	177	2.4	5.4	8.2	41.4	23.7	53.2
Orange sherbet	99	0.6	2.3	1.5	13.4	20.9	84.3
Daiquiri ice	84	-	-	-	-	20.9	100.0
Frozen yogurt: Chilled fruit salad	96	3.2	13.4	1.1	10.0	18.3	76.6
For chocolate lovers	105	4.0	15.5	1.8	15.4	18.0	69.1

BURGER CHEF

When the first Burger Chef opened its doors in Indianapolis in 1954, the customers were supposed to admire the grills as well as the food. It was a showcase for a restaurant equipment company. A quarter century later the single exhibition unit had blossomed into a chain of about 850. But Burger Chef still clings to its Midwestern roots. Most units are in Indiana and neighboring states of the heartland.

Burger Chef calculates that each outlet makes 800 sales during an average 12-hour day and that the best-selling item is the Top Shef Sandwich. It packs together a third of a pound of beef (5.3 ounces), cheese, and bacon for a caloric total of 661. More modestly caloric—and incidentally close behind in the sales column—is the Super Shef Sandwich. Built around a quarter pound of beef, it is topped with cheese, lettuce, tomato, onions, pickles, and ketchup (563 calories). Even more eclectic is the Big Shef Sandwich, which parks two burger patties (3.2 ounces of meat) under cheese, lettuce, and—here's the twist—tartar sauce, usually seen only in fish sandwiches. Calorie total: 569.

For the less adventurous, there are standard hamburgers and cheeseburgers. Fans of the latter will appreciate the double cheeseburger, whose two patties and two cheese slices amount to 420 calories—a good deal less than the special sandwiches. For dessert, there is a deep-fried apple pie, served hot. It puts a 400-calorie dent in your day.

A do-it-yourself Works Bar offers almost anything that can be dribbled, poured, or spread on a sandwich or burger. But the dieter should approach it selectively. Items with numbing calorie counts are the tartar sauce (about 75 per tablespoon) and the salad dressings (60 to 80 calories per tablespoon).

A different type of bar, the all-you-can-eat salad bar, should be the high point for dieters at Burger Chef. It features cherry tomatoes and other low-calorie items to dampen your appetite before launching into the main dishes. Croutons should be avoided, but the bacon-flavored bits, if applied judiciously, add zest at the cost of only 24 calories per tablespoon.

This is how a day with a stop at Burger Chef might look:

	Calories
BREAKFAST	
1/4 of 5-inch cantaloupe	30
1/2 cup granola with	196
1/2 cup plain, low-fat yogurt	75
Coffee or tea	0
	301
LUNCH AT BURGER CHEF:	
Hamburger (comes with ketchup, mustard, pickles;	244
add tomato and onions from Works Bar)	15

	Calories
Salad (from salad bar):	60
1 1/2 cups salad greens	
6 cherry tomatoes	
1/4 cup beets	
2 teaspoons Bac-O Bits	
1 tablespoon *(only)* blue cheese dressing	75
Coffee or tea	0
	394

DINNER:

1 cup Manhattan clam chowder	75
4 ounces broiled or baked swordfish	132
1/2 cup cooked lima beans	89
1/2 cup cooked carrots	23
1 cup mixed salad greens with vinegar or lemon juice	20
3 medium Kadota figs (water packed)	50
Coffee or tea	0
	389

SNACK:

1 cup skim milk	88

TOTAL CALORIES FOR DAY = 1,172

BURGER CHEF

Item	Calories	Protein		Fat		Carbohydrate	
		grams	% calories	grams	% calories	grams	% calories
Regular hamburger	244	11.5	19.0	8.9	33.0	29.1	48.0
Cheeseburger	290	14.4	19.9	12.6	39.5	29.3	40.6
Double Cheeseburger	420	24.3	23.4	22.3	48.2	29.5	28.4
Big Shef®	569	23.2	16.3	35.9	56.9	38.1	26.8
Super Shef®	563	29.3	20.9	29.6	47.5	44.3	31.6
TOP Shef®	661	40.5	24.9	38.1	52.7	36.4	22.4
Regular Fries	250	2.4	3.8	18.6	65.2	19.9	31.0
Large Fries	351	3.4	3.8	26.0	65.2	27.8	31.0
Fish Fillet (sandwich)	547	21.3	15.6	30.8	50.9	45.6	33.5
Mariner® Platter (two batter dipped fish fillets, fries, salad)	734	29.0	15.8	34.0	41.6	78.3	42.6

BURGER CHEF (continued)

Item	Calories	Protein		Fat		Carbohydrate	
		grams	% calories	grams	% calories	grams	% calories
Rancher® Platter (5.3 oz. beef, Texas toast, fries, salad)	640	32.4	20.2	42.2	59.2	33.1	20.6
Salad (3.5 oz.)	18	1.0	18.7	0.1	5.0	4.1	76.3
FUNMEAL® Platter	545	14.6	10.6	29.8	48.9	55.4	40.5
Hot Cocoa	198	8.3	16.5	8.2	36.8	23.4	46.7
Vanilla Shake	380	13.1	13.6	10.3	24.0	60.4	62.4
Chocolate Shake	403	10.4	10.1	9.2	20.0	72.0	69.9
Apple pie (4 oz.)*	400	2.9	2.9	24.8	55.8	41.3	41.3
Salad bar items:							
Croutons (1 oz.)	130	2.9	8.8	6.0	41.0	16.5	50.2
Cherry tomatoes (1 oz.)	6	0.3	17.7	0.05	6.4	1.3	75.9
Garbanzo beans (1 oz.)	102	5.8	22.2	1.4	11.7	17.3	66.1
Green peppers (1 oz.)	6	0.3	18.8	0.05	6.2	1.4	75.0
Shoestring beets (2 oz.)	18	0.6	12.9	0.05	2.3	4.1	84.8
Parmesan cheese (1 tbs.)	25	2.4	36.8	1.7	59.9	0.2	3.3
American cheese (1 tbs.)	21	1.3	23.5	1.8	74.8	0.1	1.7

*Calculated by authors on basis of weight provided by Burger Chef.

BURGER KING

Burger King, McDonald's chief rival in the competition to satisfy the world-wide craving for burgers, has come a long way to the Number 2 spot. In 1954 there was only a single outlet, in Miami, Florida. Today there are about 2,500 in all 50 states as well as Burger Kings in locales as diverse as the Bahamas and Hong Kong.

The company's domestic and international fortunes have been closely tied to the flagship product, the Whopper, in its various incarnations. The essential Whopper formula is a beef patty combined with lettuce, tomato, onions, pickles, ketchup, and mayonnaise. The basic formula can be varied upward to the grandiose Whopper Doublemeat with cheese, which uses two meat patties and provides almost 1,000 calories. Those who are not in need of quite so much food energy can move down to the regular Whopper (631). But for dieters, the best choice would be the Whopper Junior (369), which has a smaller patty. If you ask for the Whopper Junior without mayonnaise, you'll save 50 to 75 calories. Try using ketchup and mustard together as a substitute for the heavier topping.

Onion rings are offered as well as french fries. Dieters should note that in the regular size, the rings have 57 calories more than the fries because of their larger surface area and a coating that tends to absorb more frying oil (52 percent of the calories in the rings are from fat versus 48 percent in the fries).

While many chains provide high chairs for pint-sized patrons, some Burger King outlets go even further to equip the youngster. The high chair tray holds a paper drinking cup, bib, and pre-moistened towelette (each bearing the portrait of the bearded symbol of the chain, the Burger King himself) covered with plastic wrap. The towelette is especially useful for cleaning up child artists' finger painting, executed in ketchup.

Here's a day with lunch at Burger King. The tomato and cantaloupe at dinner both help bolster the day's vitamin A total.

	Calories
BREAKFAST:	
1/2 fresh grapefruit	55
1 large shredded wheat biscuit with	90
3/4 cup skim milk	66
	211
LUNCH AT BURGER KING:	
Whopper Junior	369
Regular french fries	209
Coffee	0
	578
DINNER:	
6 ounces broiled flounder with lemon	120
1/2 medium grilled tomato with herbs	33
1/2 cup green beans	23
1 slice whole wheat bread with	65
1/2 teaspoon margarine	17
1 1/2 cups lettuce with	12
1 tablespoon low-calorie salad dressing	15
1/6 of 5-inch cantaloupe	20
Coffee or tea	0
	305
SNACK:	
1 cup skim milk	88

TOTAL CALORIES FOR DAY = 1,182

BURGER KING®

Item	Calories	Protein		Fat		Carbohydrate	
		grams	% calories	grams	% calories	grams	% calories
Hamburger	293	15.1	20.7	12.9	39.7	29.0	39.6
Doublemeat hamburger	413	24.5	23.8	22.0	48.1	28.9	28.1
Doublemeat hamburger with cheese	519	30.3	23.4	30.8	53.5	30.0	23.1
Hamburger with cheese	347	17.9	20.6	17.4	45.2	29.6	34.2
WHOPPER Jr. Doublemeat with cheese	543	27.9	20.6	33.8	56.0	31.8	23.4
WHOPPER Jr.	369	15.4	16.7	20.2	49.3	31.3	34.0
WHOPPER Jr. Doublemeat	488	25.1	20.6	29.2	53.9	31.2	25.5
WHOPPER Jr. with cheese	424	18.3	17.2	24.7	52.5	32.0	30.3
WHOPPER	631	26.4	16.7	36.2	51.6	50.0	31.7
WHOPPER with cheese	740	31.9	17.3	45.2	54.9	51.3	27.8
WHOPPER Doublemeat with cheese	951	49.6	20.8	60.8	57.6	51.3	21.6
WHOPPER Doublemeat	843	43.9	20.8	51.9	55.5	50.0	23.7
Apple pie	250	2.9	4.6	12.5	44.8	31.6	50.6
Onion rings							
Regular	266	3.5	5.3	15.3	51.9	28.5	42.8
Large	331	4.0	4.8	19.0	51.7	36.0	43.5
French fries							
Regular	209	2.8	5.4	11.1	47.7	24.5	46.9
Large	359	5.0	5.6	19.0	47.6	42.0	46.8
Chocolate shake	337	9.2	10.9	9.7	25.9	53.2	63.2
Vanilla shake	336	9.9	11.8	10.0	26.8	51.5	61.4

CARL'S JR.

Carl's Jr. blends fast food and West Coast lifestyle at more than 240 outlets. One outlet, in Davis, California, distributes free bicycle reflectors to free-wheeling customers who order at the unusual bike-up window. There are two advantages to this: (1) you can order and eat without worrying about bicycle thieves and (2) reflectors are low in calories. Why doesn't someone invent a similar service, with mobile window, so that joggers can indulge without breaking stride?

The chain is one of the few that delivers food to your table and hands out nutritional information in the restaurant upon request. The list of calories in the leaflet is sobering to the dieter, but halfway through it you discover the salad bar—a boon if you stay clear of the thousand island and blue cheese dressing as well as the bacon bits. Substitute the Italian dressing, which has a mere 12 calories per tablespoon.

The menu reflects a characteristic California preoccupation: Each of the burgers is—what else?—a "star." The Super Star is photogenic but, at 660 calories, hardly worth the admiration of the dieter. The Famous Star and Old Time Star bring you down from the firmament into the 440's. And the Happy Star happily contains only 290, which is manageable. Although the carrot cake sounds like a dish from a health food cookbook, no one should be lulled into thinking that it is low in calories. It has more than the Happy Star or even a non-health-oriented shake.

The meal plan below shows you how to get through the day with a stop at Carl's Jr. for lunch. The salad complements the burger by adding vitamins A and C as well as folacin.

	Calories
BREAKFAST:	
3/4 cup tomato juice	35
1 poached egg on	88
1 slice whole wheat toast	65
1/2 cup skim milk	44
Coffee or tea	0
	232
LUNCH AT CARL'S JR.:	
Happy Star hamburger with	290
1 slice cheese	40
11 ounces regular salad with 1 tablespoon low-cal Italian dressing	150
Iced tea	0
	480
DINNER:	
1 5-ounce pork chop: trim off visible fat, marinate in 1/2 cup teriyaki sauce, and broil	183
2 stalks of broccoli with	64
1 tablespoon parmesan cheese	21

	Calories
1 cup cooked cauliflower	28
1 slice whole wheat bread	65
1 cup skim milk	88
Coffee or tea	0
	449

SNACK:

| 1/2 cup fresh strawberries | 27 |

TOTAL CALORIES FOR DAY = 1,188

CARL'S JR

Item	Calories	Protein		Fat		Carbohydrate	
		grams	% calories	grams	% calories	grams	% calories
Famous Star hamburger	480	27	22.4	26	48.5	35	29.1
Super Star hamburger	660	42	25.2	36	48.5	44	26.3
Old Time Star hamburger	440	26	24.0	18	37.3	42	38.7
Happy Star hamburger	290	17	23.4	11	34.0	31	42.6
Steak sandwich	630	30	19.0	28	39.9	65	41.1
California roast beef sandwich	380	30	31.4	10	23.6	43	45.0
Fish fillet sandwich	550	20	14.5	26	42.5	59	42.9
Original hot dog	340	14	16.5	19	50.5	28	33.0
Chili dog	360	17	19.0	17	42.9	34	38.1
Chili cheese dog	400	19	19.0	20	45.0	36	36.0
American cheese slice	40	3	27.9	3	62.8	1	9.3
11-oz. regular salad with condiments	170	8	19.6	3	16.6	26	63.8

CARL'S JR. (continued)

Item	Calories	Protein		Fat		Carbohydrate	
		grams	% calories	grams	% calories	grams	% calories
4 tbs. blue cheese dressing	200	4	8.6	19	91.4	-	-
4 tbs. thousand island dressing	190	1	2.1	18	87.1	5	10.8
4 tbs. low-cal Italian dressing	48	-	-	-	-	1	100.0
French fries Regular (3 oz.)	220	4	7.3	8	32.7	33	60.0
Big scoop (4 oz.)	293	5	7.3	12	32.7	43	60.0
Onion rings	320	5	6.2	18	50.3	35	43.5
Apple turnover	330	4	4.9	15	41.3	44	53.8
Carrot cake	380	5	5.5	18	44.2	46	50.3
Shakes (20-oz. cup)	310	14	15.8	7	17.7	59	66.5

CHURCH'S FRIED CHICKEN

A subcategory of Southern fried chicken is Southwestern fried chicken, the style at Church's, a Texas-based chain of almost 1,000 outlets. The hallmark is the jalapeño pepper that comes with some dinners and can be ordered a la carte by aficionados of the fiery condiment. Also, the trimmings are kept to a select few: cole slaw, french fries, corn on the cob, and pecan or apple pie.

Church's has resolved a long-standing dining dilemma: how to eat corn on the cob, dripping with butter, without looking like a slob. The answer is simple. Put it on a stick and eat it like ice cream. It's a particularly handy method for take-out customers, who are Church's mainstay.

Dieters should plan to eat at Church's for dinner, since the basic meal is rather large. The Chicken Snack consists of a big piece of poultry (316 calories) plus a roll (83). Round out the meal with the 3-ounce serving of cole slaw (123) and the corn on the cob (165).

The meal plan below shows you how to incorporate the dinner in your day's eating. The breakfast is light, to allow for the corn at dinner, but it does have a fortified cereal with milk to help fulfill the daily need for calcium, iron, zinc, and magnesium. There is also a way to increase your vitamin intake: Eat the peppers. They are only 4 calories each and are rich in vitamins A and C.

	Calories

BREAKFAST:

1 1/2 cups Special K cereal with	105
1/2 cup skim milk	44
Coffee or tea	0
	149

LUNCH:

3/4 cup tomato juice	35
1 cup low-fat cottage cheese with chives	176
1 sliced medium tomato	33
1 sliced cucumber (unpeeled)	16
1 sliced small green pepper	16
2 1/4 cups lettuce	18
1 slice whole wheat bread	65
Iced tea with lemon	0
	359

DINNER AT CHURCH'S:

Chicken Snack:	
1 piece chicken	316
1 roll	83
Cole slaw	123
Corn on the cob	165
Jalapeño pepper	4
Coffee or tea	0
	691

TOTAL CALORIES FOR DAY = 1,199

CHURCH'S FRIED CHICKEN

Item	Calories	Protein grams	Protein % calories	Fat grams	Fat % calories	Carbohydrate grams	Carbohydrate % calories
Chicken Snack:							
Chicken (l large piece)	316	20.2	25.4	22.1	62.8	9.3	11.8
Dinner roll* (1 oz.)	83	2.3	11.1	1.6	17.4	14.8	71.5

CHURCH'S FRIED CHICKEN (continued)

Item	Calories	Protein		Fat		Carbohydrate	
		grams	% calories	grams	% calories	grams	% calories
French fries* (3 oz.)	256	3.8	6.0	12.8	45.0	31.3	49.0
Corn on the cob* (9 oz., buttered)	165	4.5	10.9	3.3	18.1	29.2	70.9
Jalapeño pepper*	4	0.1	10.8	0.01	2.4	0.8	86.7
Pecan Pie* (3 oz.)	367	4.4	4.8	19.5	47.8	43.6	47.5
Apple pie* (3 oz.)	300	2.2	2.9	18.6	55.8	31.0	41.3
Cole slaw* (3 oz.)	83	1.0	4.5	7.0	68.3	6.0	27.0

*Calculated on the basis of weights provided by Church's.

DAIRY QUEEN

Perhaps the best tribute to Dairy Queen's salesmanship is that it manages to sell frozen dessert in Alaska. Its half dozen stands in that state are part of a far-flung empire embracing almost 5,000 outlets. Texans seem especially fond of the red-roofed stands. The Lone Star State keeps almost 1,000 of them in business. The chain has shown its appreciation by offering only that state a Texas-sized burger called the Belt Buster. But other states still enjoy a wide variety of burgers, hot dogs, fish sandwiches, and desserts.

For the dieter, a big advantage at Dairy Queen is the variable-size portions. A full-size model, for example, is the Triple Burger with cheese, which adds 840 calories to your day. But you can scale down by choosing one of the lower orders of magnitude, like the Double Burger (540) or the demure Single Burger (370).

The Chili Dog is a pastiche. Atop a conventional hot dog and bun are piled chili (with ground beef and beans), mustard, and relish. Delicate it's not, but it does satisfy a hearty hunger, and for a relatively bearable 330 calories.

Of course, few can tear themselves away without at least a small sample of the firm's original product, so the day shown below is punctuated by a Dairy Queen lunch with dessert. The vanilla cone provides a nutritional bonus in the form of calcium (NDS = 216).

	Calories

BREAKFAST:

1 cup Puffed Rice cereal with	51
1/2 cup fresh or frozen blueberries (unsweetened) and	24
3/4 cup skim milk	66
Coffee or tea	0
	141

LUNCH AT DAIRY QUEEN:

Chili Dog	330
Small vanilla cone	110
Coffee or tea	0
	440

DINNER:

6-ounce broiled flank steak (well trimmed):	301
marinated and baste with 2 tablespoons Worcester-	
shire sauce, 2 tablespoons chopped onion, 1 tablespoon	
tomato juice, 1/2 tablespoon grated fresh ginger	
1 small (5-ounce) baked potato with	106
2 tablespoons plain, low-fat yogurt and chives	16
2/3 cup peas	71
1 shredded, small carrot cooked with	45
1/4 cup diced pineapple (water-packed or fresh)	
1/4 of 5-inch honeydew melon (or 1 cup frozen	33
melon balls) with wedge of lemon	
Coffee or tea	0
	572

SNACK:

Late-night crunchies:	30
1 cup raw string beans	

TOTAL CALORIES FOR DAY = 1,183

DAIRY QUEEN

Item	Calories	Protein		Fat		Carbohydrate	
		grams	% calories	grams	% calories	grams	% calories
Burgers							
Single	370	20	22.2	16	40.0	34	37.8
Single with cheese	470	27	23.3	24	46.5	35	30.2

DAIRY QUEEN (continued)

Item	Calories	Protein		Fat		Carbohydrate	
		grams	% calories	grams	% calories	grams	% calories
Double	540	35	26.1	29	48.6	34	25.3
Double with cheese	650	42	26.2	37	52.0	35	21.8
Triple	740	51	27.8	42	51.5	38	20.7
Triple with cheese	840	57	27.3	50	54.0	39	18.7
Brazier Cheese Dog	330	15	18.3	19	52.3	24	29.4
Brazier Chili Dog	330	13	15.7	20	54.2	25	30.1
Brazier Dog	273	11	16.2	15	49.8	23	34.0
French fries (2.5 oz.)	200	2	4.0	10	45.5	25	50.5
(4 oz.)	320	3	3.8	16	45.6	40	50.6
Onion rings	300	6	7.8	17	49.5	33	42.7
Fish sandwich	400	20	20.2	17	38.5	41	41.3
Fish sandwich with cheese	440	24	21.8	21	42.8	39	35.4
Super Brazier Dog	518	20	15.6	30	52.5	41	31.9
Super Brazier Dog with cheese	593	26	17.3	36	54.0	43	28.7
Super Brazier Chili Dog	555	23	16.5	33	53.3	42	30.2
Banana split	540	10	7.4	15	25.0	91	67.5
Buster Bar	390	10	10.4	22	51.3	37	38.3
Chocolate dipped cone small	150	3	7.8	7	40.6	20	51.6
medium	300	7	9.2	13	38.4	40	52.4
large	450	10	8.9	20	39.8	58	51.3
Chocolate malt small	340	10	11.6	11	28.9	51	59.5
medium	600	15	10.1	20	30.2	89	59.7
large	840	22	10.5	28	30.0	125	59.5
Chocolate sundae small	170	4	9.3	4	20.9	30	69.8
medium	300	6	8.0	7	21.1	53	70.9
large	400	9	9.0	9	20.2	71	70.8

DAIRY QUEEN (continued)

Item	Calories	Protein		Fat		Carbohydrate	
		grams	% calories	grams	% calories	grams	% calories
Plain cone							
small	110	3	10.8	3	24.3	18	64.9
medium	230	6	10.6	7	27.7	35	61.7
large	340	10	11.8	10	26.6	52	61.6
Parfait	460	10	8.6	11	21.4	81	70.0
Dilly Bar	240	4	6.7	15	56.5	22	36.8
Float	330	6	7.2	8	21.7	59	71.1
Freeze	520	11	8.5	13	22.6	89	68.9
Sandwich	140	3	8.3	4	25.0	24	66.7
Hot fudge brownie delight	570	11	7.7	22	34.5	83	57.8
Mr. Misty float	440	6	5.5	8	16.5	85	78.0
Mr. Misty freeze	500	10	8.1	12	21.8	87	70.1

DUNKIN' DONUTS SHOPS

Dunkin' Donuts has spread the donut-eating culture from the United States to Japan, where the beige and pink packages of take-out pastries are helping to balance the trade deficit caused by our overindulgence in small cars and color televisions.

If your food fantasy is to imagine yourself at the end of your local Dunkin' Donuts Shop's assembly line, devouring a chocolate-covered donut here and a yeast-raised donut there, you probably wish that you were a 90-pound weakling in dire need of calories.

While dieting, the only part of the donut that is safe to eat is the hole. Luckily, Dunkin' Donuts thought so too and invented Munchkins, which are essentially just that. The little round pastries come in all the regular flavors, but only the yeast-raised type (with no filling) are relatively modest in calories. Consider them a special treat.

You can work a Dunkin' Donuts break into your day like this:

	Calories
BREAKFAST:	
Apricot eye-opener:	265
2 tablespoons grapenuts cereal	
2/3 cup 100% Bran Flakes	

	Calories
1/2 cup plain, low-fat yogurt (or 3/4 cup skim milk)	
5 dried apricot halves	
Coffee or tea	0
	265

LUNCH:

California sandwich:	253
1 slice cracked wheat bread	
2 tablespoons low-fat cream cheese (Neufchatel)	
1/3 sliced cucumber (unpeeled)	
1/4 sliced avocado	
1/4 cup alfalfa sprouts	
1/2 sliced medium tomato	
1 cup skim milk	88
	341

AFTERNOON TREAT AT DUNKIN' DONUTS:

6 yeast-raised Munchkins (2 with glaze)	176
Coffee or tea	0
	176

DINNER:

3 ounces baked ham:	
glazed with 1 teaspoon frozen orange juice	173
concentrate	
1 small baked sweet potato	148
1 cup French-style string beans with	31
1/2 cup sliced mushrooms (fresh)	5
1 small orange	49
Coffee or tea	0
	406

TOTAL CALORIES FOR DAY = 1,188

DUNKIN' DONUTS SHOPS*

Item	Calories*	Protein		Fat		Carbohydrate	
		grams	% calories	grams	% calories	grams	% calories
Cake and chocolate cake donuts (include rings, sticks, crullers, etc.)	240	2.9	4.8	11.4	42.8	31.5	52.5

DUNKIN' DONUTS SHOPS* (continued)

Item	Calories*	Protein		Fat		Carbohydrate	
		grams	% calories	grams	% calories	grams	% calories
Yeast-raised donuts	160	2.5	2.5	10.3	57.8	14.5	36.4
(add 5-10 calories for glaze)							
(add 40-50 calories for filling and topping combined)							
Munchkins							
Cake and chocolate cake	66	0.8	4.8	3.1	42.8	8.7	52.5
Yeast-raised	26	0.4	6.1	1.7	57.8	2.4	36.4
(add 10-15 calories for filling, and topping combined)							
Fancies (includes coffee rolls, danish, etc.)	215	3.7	7.2	10.0	47.8	23.3	45.0

*Caloric values provided by Dunkin' Donuts Shops; composition calculated using USDA Handbook No. 8.

FRIENDLY RESTAURANTS

Friendly has grown from an old-fashioned soda fountain into a family restaurant. The chain dates back to July 1935, when a pair of brothers in Springfield, Massachusetts, opened a shop offering double-dip ice cream cones at 5 cents each. They chose the name Friendly to symbolize the ambience they hoped to create.

When winter arrived, burgers were added to keep the customers' interest. The french fries, though, didn't arrive for another 30 years. By then, the chain was well on its way toward its present total of over 600 restaurants, stretching from New England south to the mid-Atlantic states and west to the Mississippi. Friendly now provides booths as well as counter service and full-meal offerings. It is expanding its menu to include such favorites as veal Parmesan.

For many the ice cream and fountain creations are still the highlight. The deluxe model is the Jim Dandy (925 calories), four scoops of ice cream, a banana, nuts, strawberry, chocolate, marshmallow, and whipped toppings. The vanilla Fribble, an extra-thick shake (620), and the Fribble Junior (450) are similarly tempting.

One possible strategy for dieters is to compromise on a simple ice cream as a special treat, perhaps indulging yourself with 34 extra calories worth of chocolate sprinkles. The following meal plan shows you how to do it without exceeding your daily calorie limit. The wheat germ at breakfast provides a bonus in the form of B vitamins and vitamin E.

	Calories
BREAKFAST:	
3/4 cup unsweetened grapefruit juice	66
3/4 cup oatmeal with	88
1 tablespoon raisins and	29
1 tablespoon wheat germ	23
1/2 cup skim milk	44
Coffe or tea	0
	250
LUNCH:	
3/4 cup three-bean salad	143
1/4 cup low-fat cottage cheese	45
1 medium orange	73
Coffee or tea	0
	261
TREAT AT FRIENDLY:	
1 regular scoop of vanilla ice cream with sugar cone	290
DINNER:	
3/4 cup tomato juice	35
4 ounces sea bass baked with lemon and fresh parsley	110
1/2 cup peas and carrots	52
1/2 cup whole boiled potatoes with	59
1/2 teaspoon margarine and parsley	17
1 slice whole wheat bread	65
1 cup mixed greens with lemon juice or vinegar	20
Coffee or tea	0
	358
SNACK:	
1/2 cup fresh strawberries	27

TOTAL CALORIES FOR DAY = 1,186

FRIENDLY

Item	Calories	Protein		Fat		Carbohydrate	
		grams	% calories	grams	% calories	grams	% calorie
Hamburger with roll and butter	370	25.0	27.0	18.0	43.8	27.0	29.2
Big Beef with bread, butter, and pickles	450	35.2	32.1	22.0	45.1	25.0	22.8
Friendly Frank with roll and butter	370	11.8	12.7	24.0	58.2	27.0	29.1
Ice cream cones							
Sugar cones							
Regular (4 oz.)							
Vanilla	290	4.0	5.4	14.0	42.9	38.0	51.7
Chocolate	310	5.0	6.5	14.0	40.6	41.0	52.9
Double Dip (7 oz.)							
Vanilla	460	7.0	6.1	23.0	44.7	57.0	49.2
Chocolate	488	8.0	6.3	24.0	44.3	63.0	49.4
Cake Cones							
Regular (4 oz.)							
Vanilla	248	4.0	6.4	13.0	47.0	29.0	46.6
Chocolate	262	5.0	7.5	13.0	44.2	32.0	48.3
Double dip (7 oz.)							
Vanilla	420	7.0	6.6	22.0	46.9	49.0	46.5
Chocolate	444	8.0	7.1	23.0	45.5	53.9	47.4
Chocolate sprinkles (¼ oz.)	34	-	-	2.0	60.0	4.0	40.0
Ice cream sundae (vanilla ice cream)							
Hot fudge	590	9.0	6.1	28.0	42.9	75.0	51.0
Strawberry	420	6.0	5.7	20.0	42.9	54.0	51.4
Fudge Royal	770	11.0	5.7	38.0	44.2	97.0	50.1
Jim Dandy	925	12.0	5.1	40.0	38.1	134.0	56.8
Strawberry Royal	590	8.0	5.3	30.0	44.9	75.0	49.8
Milk Shakes							
Vanilla	520	16.0	12.3	21.0	36.3	67.0	51.4
Chocolate	617	16.0	10.4	22.0	32.0	89.0	57.6

Item	Calories	Protein		Fat		Carbohydrate	
		grams	% calories	grams	% calories	grams	% calories

FRIENDLY (continued)

Item	Calories	grams	% calories	grams	% calories	grams	% calories
Fribble							
Vanilla	620	24.0	15.5	17.0	24.6	93.0	59.9
Vanilla-Junior	450	15.0	13.4	10.0	20.2	74.0	66.4
Chocolate	670	25.0	14.5	18.0	23.5	107.0	62.0

NOTE: The nutritional information in this chart has been developed by Friendly Restaurants from published tables based on the average composition of foods and not on actual analysis. Friendly makes no nutritional claims for its food and offers the information only as a guide in meal planning.

GINO'S

Gino's is a chain that sticks close to home. Although it has 350 outlets, almost all of them are in the Philadelphia-Baltimore-Washington, D.C., area. (It's even named for a local football star—former tight end Gino Marchetti of the Baltimore Colts.) But what it lacks in geographical diversity, the chain makes up in menu variety. It serves a full line of burgers and sandwiches. What's more, if you've recently eaten a meal at Kentucky Fried Chicken, walking into Gino's can give you a strong sense of *déjà vu*. That's because Gino's acts as a franchise for the Colonel's favorite dish in a large segment of the mid-Atlantic area. In sum, the Gino's bill of fare might be described as "finger lickin' burgers."

Two main items are the Giant and the Sirloiner. The Giant, a double burger with mayonnaise-type dressing, pickle, and lettuce, weighs in at 569 calories. The Sirloiner combines a quarter pound of sirloin with onions, pickle, ketchup, and mustard for 436 calories. The Home-style hamburger (513) is a quarter pounder on a roll that allows you to exercise your imagination by adding anything you want from the salad bar.

The dieter's best strategy is to make ample use of the extensive salad bar to create a large, satisfying yet reasonable meal that's adequate in vitamins A and C. Make it a major meal of the day, in this fashion:

	Calories
BREAKFAST:	
1 sliced medium orange	73
1 poached egg on	88
1 slice whole wheat toast	65
Coffee or tea	0
	226

	Calories

LUNCH AT GINO'S:

1 serving of salad from salad bar: 75
    take a lot of lettuce and a variety of other ingredients;
    go easy on the cheese, Bac-O Bits, chick peas; instead
    of dressing use lemon juice, salt, and pepper

Sirloiner   436

Coffee or tea   0

                                               511

DINNER:

1 large celery stalk   10

4 ounce baked or broiled halibut steak served with wedge   192
    of lemon

1 cup of broccoli   40

Oven baked chips: 106
    peel a small (5-ounce) potato, cut into wedges as for
    french fries; place on cookie sheet sprayed with Pam
    or other nonstick spray, bake at 425° for 30 to 40
    minutes until brown

1 tablespoon ketchup   24

Coffee or tea   0

                                               372

SNACK:

3/4 cup skim milk   66

TOTAL CALORIES FOR DAY = 1,175

GINO'S

Item	Calories	Protein		Fat		Carbohydrate	
		grams	% calories	grams	% calories	grams	% calories
Hamburger	249	11.3	17.7	8.8	31.1	32.6	51.2
Cheeseburger	295	14.2	18.8	12.5	37.2	33.2	44.0
Sirloiner	436	23.8	21.9	21.7	44.9	36.2	33.2
Cheese Sirloiner	526	29.5	22.4	29.1	49.8	36.6	27.8
Giant	569	22.0	15.5	32.7	51.8	46.4	32.7
Home-style hamburger	513	31.9	25.5	28.0	50.3	30.4	24.3
Roast beef	413	29.7	29.1	17.0	37.4	34.2	33.5
Cheese steak	496	32.7	26.2	24.7	44.5	36.7	29.3

GINO'S (continued)

Item	Calories	Protein		Fat		Carbohydrate	
		grams	% calories	grams	% calories	grams	% calories
Fish sandwich	445	12.4	11.8	25.6	55.1	34.6	33.1
Fish platter	650	18.0	10.9	43.0	58.6	50.3	30.5
French fries	172	2.6	5.9	8.2	42.3	22.6	51.8
Milk shakes							
Vanilla	310	17.3	22.3	9.5	27.6	38.8	50.1
Chocolate	324	19.4	25.0	9.7	28.1	36.4	46.8
Mini Desserts							
Chocolate	250	3.0	4.8	14.0	50.4	28.0	44.8
Strawberry	210	2.0	3.8	8.0	34.6	32.0	61.6
Cheesecake	210	6.0	11.2	10.0	42.1	25.0	46.7
Salad bar items:							
Lettuce (2 oz.)	7	0.5	23.8	-	-	1.6	76.2
Onions (1 oz.)	11	0.4	13.8	-	-	2.5	86.2
Tomato (2 oz.)	13	0.6	17.0	0.1	6.4	2.7	76.6
Cucumbers (½ oz.)	2	0.1	16.7	-	-	0.5	83.3
Radishes (¾ oz.)	4	0.2	20.0	-	-	0.8	80.0
Celery (½ oz.)	2	0.1	14.3	-	-	0.6	85.7
Carrots (¼ oz.)	3	0.1	12.5	-	-	0.7	87.5
Kidney beans (1 oz.)	26	1.6	24.9	0.1	3.5	4.6	71.6
Chick peas (1 oz.)	102	5.8	22.1	1.4	12.0	17.3	65.9
Beets (1 oz.)	10	0.3	10.7	-	-	2.5	89.3
Green beans (1 oz.)	7	0.4	18.8	0.1	10.6	1.5	70.6
Peperoncini (½ oz.)	5	0.2	13.3	-	-	1.3	86.7
Bean sprouts (1 oz.)	8	0.9	34.3	0.1	8.6	1.5	57.1
Bac-O Bits (¼ oz.)	29	2.8	38.4	1.2	37.0	1.8	24.6
Grated cheese food (¼ oz.)	28	2.6	38.0	1.8	59.1	0.2	2.9
Green peppers (¾ oz.)	5	0.2	16.7	-	-	1.0	83.3
Dressings (1 tbs.)							
Italian	60	-	-	7.0	94.0	1.0	6.0

GINO'S (continued)

Item	Calories	Protein		Fat		Carbohydrate	
		grams	% calories	grams	% calories	grams	% calories
French	60	-	-	6.0	87.1	2.0	12.9
Russian	60	-	-	6.0	87.1	2.0	12.9
Bleu cheese	80	1.0	5.3	8.0	94.7	-	-

In some Gino's outlets Kentucky Fried Chicken is also sold. See Kentucky Fried Chicken char for nutrition information.

HARDEE'S

Once a basic-burger operation, Hardee's underwent a face lift in the lat 1970's. The architecture was redesigned, more drive-through windows wer added, and the menu was expanded. Even the old regular burger patty wa transformed—beefed up by 25 percent to match the bolder image.

Although fast food is often blamed for obliterating regional cooking, par of Hardee's plan is the resurrection of an old Southern favorite, the biscui breakfast. It's available below the Mason-Dixon line, where about half o Hardee's 1,200 outlets are found.

The biscuits (275 calories each) are billed as homemade and can be com bined with sausage, steak, ham, or egg. The complete breakfast ranges from ; high of 527 calories for the steak-biscuit-egg combination to 349 for the biscui with ham. Choosing sausage instead of ham raises the calorie total by 64 anc makes the dish considerably higher in fat (57 percent of calories versus 4 percent). Those watching their sodium intake should be aware that each biscui contains 650 mg.

Hardee's also offers a roast beef sandwich (390 calories) and a big versio of it that improves the beef-to-bun ratio but adds 95 calories. The ham anc cheese sandwich (376) is served hot. Besides the new, improved burger (305) there is an even larger Deluxe. It combines a quarter pound patty with tomato onion, lettuce, and a mayonnaise-based sauce for a grand total of 675 calories— the most caloric item on the menu.

Here's how to spend a day, beginning with a breakfast at Hardee's:

	Calories
BREAKFAST AT HARDEE'S:	
3/4 cup orange juice	90
Ham biscuit	349
Coffee or tea	0
	439

	Calories

LUNCH:

1 sliced small banana with	85
1 cup plain, low-fat yogurt and dash cinnamon	130
Coffee or tea	0
	215

DINNER:

3/4 cup tomato juice	35
4 ounces barbecued or broiled veal steak: marinate in lemon juice, garlic, and pepper	179
1/2 cup green beans	23
1/2 cup mashed winter squash	38
1 slice whole wheat bread	65
1 cup mixed salad greens with	20
1 tablespoon low-calorie salad dressing	15
3/4 cup fresh pineapple (or 1 large slice canned pineapple packed in juice)	55
Coffee or tea	0
	430

SNACK:

1 cup skim milk	88

TOTAL CALORIES FOR DAY = 1,172

HARDEE'S

Item	Calories	Protein		Fat		Carbohydrate	
		grams	% calories	grams	% calories	grams	% calories
Hamburger	305	16.5	21.7	13.4	39.7	29.4	38.6
Cheeseburger	335	17.2	20.6	16.8	45.2	28.7	34.2
Double cheeseburger	495	29.6	23.9	29.6	53.8	27.6	22.3
Deluxe	675	31.1	18.4	41.0	54.5	45.8	27.1
Big Twin	447	23.8	21.2	26.1	52.5	29.4	26.3
Roast beef sandwich	390	17.0	17.3	16.3	37.5	44.2	45.2
Big roast beef sandwich	485	24.8	20.5	26.1	48.5	37.6	31.0
Fish sandwich	468	16.5	14.1	26.1	50.1	41.9	35.8
Hot Ham 'n' Cheese	376	22.8	24.2	15.2	36.4	37.0	39.4

HARDEE'S (continued)

Item	Calories	Protein		Fat		Carbohydrate	
		grams	% calories	grams	% calories	grams	% calories
Hot dog	346	11.2	12.9	22.0	57.2	25.8	29.9
French fries							
Small	239	3.1	5.2	13.0	48.7	27.6	46.1
Large	381	5.0	5.2	20.6	48.7	43.8	46.1
Apple turnover	282	2.5	3.6	13.8	44.1	36.9	52.3
Milk shake	391	11.4	11.7	10.4	24.0	62.9	64.3
Biscuit	275	4.8	6.9	13.0	42.5	34.7	50.6
Ham biscuit	349	12.4	14.1	16.9	43.6	37.0	42.3
Steak biscuit	419	13.6	13.0	22.5	48.3	40.6	38.7
Sausage biscuit	413	10.1	9.8	26.3	57.3	34.0	32.9
One medium fried egg	108	6.2	23.9	8.6	74.6	0.4	1.5
Biscuit with egg	383	11.0	11.6	21.6	51.3	35.1	37.1
Ham biscuit with egg	458	18.6	16.4	25.5	50.7	37.4	33.0
Steak biscuit with egg	527	19.8	15.2	31.1	53.5	41.0	31.3
Sausage biscuit with egg	521	16.3	12.6	34.9	60.7	34.4	26.6

JACK IN THE BOX

Some chains have grown like Topsy. Jack in the Box has grown from Topsy's—a San Diego car-hop restaurant that opened its parking spaces in 1941. By 1968 the drive-in had blossomed into a 265-outlet enterprise under the Jack in the Box trademark. Today there are more than 1,000 of the restaurants, most heavily concentrated in California, Arizona, and Texas. A mini-chain of seven operates in São Paulo, Brazil.

The menu offers a variety of burger and cheeseburger combinations. The top-of-the-line model (628 calories) is the Jumbo Jack cheeseburger, a quarter-pounder with cheese, which is garnished with tomato, lettuce, relish, onion, pickle, and special sauce. Both the Hamburger Deluxe (260) and Cheeseburger Deluxe (314) come with a mayonnaise-based sauce, as well as the garnishes. The Moby Jack, a whale of a fish sandwich (455 calories), is topped with tartar sauce and cheese. "Flaked and formed" beef goes into the Jack Steak Sandich (428), along with tomato, lettuce, and steak sauce. It's served on a French ll.

Jack in the Box is one of the chains that has made a special effort to tract breakfast eaters. Your morning options include French toast, pancakes, d scrambled eggs. None of the three is below 500 calories, and the scrambled gs (with ham links, hash browns, English muffin, and jelly) comes to 719, the ghest calorie count on the entire menu. It also has a relatively high fat ntent (54.8 percent of calories).

The lowest calorie eye-opener (301) is the Breakfast Jack sandwich, a mbination of ham, egg, and cheese on a hamburger bun. But for something fferent you might try the Ranchero style omelette (414), which is made with eese and a zippy, tomato-based "salsa." The other omelettes, ham and cheese d double cheese, have about the same number of calories, but are more con- ntional. An English muffin accompanies all omelettes.

Below is a day starting with a brunch at Jack in the Box. The spinach at nner bolsters the day's intake of folacin, iron, and vitamins A and C.

	Calories
BRUNCH AT JACK IN THE BOX:	
Ranchero style omelette with English muffin and jelly	414
Coffee or tea	0
	414
LUNCH:	
1 cup plain, low-fat yogurt (or	130
1 cup low-fat cottage cheese) with	(180)
1/2 cup crushed pineapple (packed in juice)	64
Iced tea	0
	194 (244)
DINNER:	
6 ounces red snapper baked with lemon	165
1/2 cup cooked spinach with dash of nutmeg and freshly ground black pepper	21
1/2 cup cooked white or brown rice: cook rice in water flavored with 1 chicken bouillon cube	85
1 slice whole wheat bread with	65
1/2 teaspoon margarine	17
1 small orange	49
Coffee or tea	0
	402

	Calories

SNACK:

Strawberry treat: 115
   mix in a blender or food processor
     1/2 cup frozen strawberries (unsweetened)
     1 cup skim milk

TOTAL CALORIES FOR DAY = 1,125 (1,175)

JACK IN THE BOX

Item	Calories	Protein		Fat		Carbohydrate	
		grams	% calories	grams	% calories	grams	% calories
Hamburger	263	12.6	19.2	10.6	36.4	29.1	44.4
Cheeseburger	310	15.6	20.1	14.9	43.3	28.3	36.6
Hamburger Deluxe	260	13.0	20.0	10.2	35.3	29.1	44.7
Cheeseburger Deluxe	314	15.1	19.2	15.1	43.2	29.5	37.6
Bonus Jack® Hamburger	461	23.9	20.7	23.5	45.9	38.5	33.4
Jumbo Jack® Hamburger	551	28.0	20.3	28.8	47.1	44.8	32.6
Jumbo Jack® Hamburger with cheese	628	32.1	20.5	35.4	50.7	45.2	28.8
Regular taco	189	7.9	16.8	10.9	52.0	14.7	31.2
Super taco	285	12.3	17.3	17.4	55.0	19.7	27.7
Jack Burrito®	448	21.2	19.0	22.0	44.2	41.2	36.8
Moby Jack® Sandwich	455	17.2	15.1	26.2	51.7	37.8	33.2
Jack steak® Sandwich	428	27.4	25.5	19.6	41.1	35.8	33.4
Breakfast Jack® Sandwich	301	17.8	23.6	13.1	39.1	28.1	37.3
French fries	270	2.9	4.3	14.9	49.7	31.0	46.0
Onion rings	351	4.7	5.4	22.7	58.2	32.0	36.4
Lemon turnover	446	4.3	3.9	25.7	51.8	49.4	44.3
Apple turnover	411	3.8	3.7	23.9	52.4	45.1	43.9

JACK IN THE BOX (continued)

Item	Calories	Protein		Fat		Carbohydrate	
		grams	% calories	grams	% calories	grams	% calories
Shake*							
Vanilla	317	9.5	11.8	6.3	17.6	56.7	70.6
Strawberry	323	10.5	13.0	6.6	18.4	55.4	68.6
Chocolate	325	10.9	13.5	6.8	18.9	54.7	67.6
Shake†							
Vanilla	342	10.0	11.7	9.4	24.7	54.0	63.2
Chocolate	365	10.5	11.5	9.5	23.4	59.3	65.0
Strawberry	380	10.5	11.1	9.5	22.5	63.0	66.3
Ham and Cheese omelette	425	21.2	20.0	23.3	49.4	32.4	30.6
Double Cheese omelette	423	19.4	18.3	24.9	53.0	30.4	28.7
Ranchero Style omelette	414	19.6	19.0	22.7	49.5	32.5	31.5
French Toast Breakfast	537	15.3	11.4	28.8	48.2	54.2	40.4
Pancakes Breakfast	626	16.2	10.3	27.4	39.4	78.7	50.3
Scrambled Eggs Breakfast	719	25.9	14.4	43.8	54.8	55.3	30.8

*Shakes sold in California, Arizona, Texas, and Washington.
†Shakes sold in all other states.

ENTUCKY FRIED CHICKEN

efore World War II, Harland Sanders was a service station operator, in Corbin, entucky, who was in the habit of feeding hungry travelers his home-cooked icken. Before long, the customers had begun dropping in for the food instead ˮ the gas and the governor had declared him an honorary Kentucky Colonel r meritorious cuisine. The Colonel's likeness became the trademark of the entucky Fried Chicken Corporation, which markets his "still-secret combina- on of 11 herbs and spices" through about 6,000 outlets.

Fried chicken has long been an American favorite, but people seem to ave strong preferences for the way they like it done. Even homespun Colonel anders opted for some academic training—at the Cornell University School of otel Administration—to perfect his technique. The result has won a wide idience, perhaps because it bridges the gap between those who like chicken ne with moderate crispness and those who like it very crisp.

The Kentucky Fried Chicken menu is based on a standard dinner, cor sisting of three pieces of chicken, a roll, mashed potato with gravy, and col slaw. The average calorie total for the dinner is 636–777 if you like it extr crispy—but there is some flexibility in the combination of chicken pieces tha can affect the calorie count. For the original dinner the wing-thigh combina tion is highest (393 for the chicken alone). The drumstick-thigh amounts t 374 and the wing-rib comes to 335. By ordering the latter, in other word: dieters save 58 calories. Better yet, order a single piece of chicken.

To many people, the crusty skin is the best part of the dish. But if you tastes are flexible enough to peel off the skin and forget about it, you ca save over 100 calories.

Even with the gravy, the mashed potatoes (86 calories) are a diet plu compared to french fries (156), and they have half the fat. To save even mor calories and fat, have the roll without the butter.

One way to build a day around dinner at Kentucky Fried Chicken i shown below. The vitamin C in the strawberries (NDS = more than 5,000 compensates for the low level of the vitamin in the dinner.

	Calories
BREAKFAST:	
1 cup Total cereal with	108
3/4 cup skim milk and	66
1/2 cup fresh or frozen strawberries (unsweetened)	27
Coffee or tea	0
	201
LUNCH:	
Good Earth salad:	175
1 cup romaine lettuce	
1/2 cup fresh spinach	
4 sliced large mushrooms (fresh)	
1/4 cup alfalfa sprouts	
1/4 cup kidney beans	
1 sliced medium tomato	
1/4 cup chick peas	
Thinly sliced Bermuda onions	
Vinegar or lemon juice	
1 slice whole wheat bread with	65
1/2 teaspoon margarine	17
1 cup skim milk	88
	345
DINNER AT KENTUCKY FRIED CHICKEN (eaten at home):	
1 piece chicken rib	199
(add 35 more calories for extra crispy)	

	Calories
Cole slaw	122
Mashed potatoes and gravy	86
Roll (order it without butter)	61
Coffee or tea	0
1/6 of 5-inch cantaloupe	20
	488

SNACK:

Blueberry yogurt freeze: 132
    Mix in blender or food processor
        1/2 cup frozen blueberries (unsweetened)
        1/2 small banana
        1/2 cup plain, low-fat yogurt
        Dash of cinnamon

      TOTAL CALORIES FOR DAY = 1,164

KENTUCY FRIED CHICKEN

Item	Calories	Protein		Fat		Carbohydrate	
		grams	% calories	grams	% calories	grams	% calories
Original Recipe Chicken							
Wing	136	9.6	28.2	9.0	59.5	4.2	12.3
Drumstick	117	12.1	41.3	6.5	49.9	2.6	8.9
Keel	235	23.9	40.5	12.3	46.9	7.4	12.5
Rib	199	16.2	32.6	11.7	53.0	7.1	14.3
Thigh	257	18.4	28.6	17.5	61.3	6.5	10.1
Extra Crispy Chicken							
Wing	201	11.2	22.3	13.5	60.4	8.7	17.3
Drumstick	155	13.3	34.4	9.0	52.4	5.1	13.2
Keel	297	23.6	31.8	16.4	49.8	13.6	18.4
Rib	286	17.2	24.1	17.8	56.1	14.1	19.8
Thigh	343	20.4	23.8	23.4	61.5	12.6	14.7
Dinner (2 pieces, roll, mashed potato/ gravy, cole slaw)							
Original Recipe							
Wing/Rib	604	30.4	20.1	32.1	47.9	48.3	32.0

KENTUCKY FRIED CHICKEN (continued)

Item	Calories	Protein		Fat		Carbohydrate	
		grams	% calories	grams	% calories	grams	% calories
Wing/Thigh	662	32.6	19.7	37.8	51.4	47.8	28.9
Drumstick/Thigh	643	35.1	21.9	35.2	49.3	46.2	28.8
Extra Crispy							
Wing/Rib	755	33.0	17.5	42.6	50.8	59.9	31.7
Wing/Thigh	812	36.2	17.8	48.2	53.4	58.4	28.8
Drumstick/Thigh	765	38.3	20.0	43.7	51.4	54.7	28.6
Roll (without butter)	61	1.8	11.9	1.1	16.3	10.9	71.8
Mashed potato and gravy	86	1.9	8.8	2.7	28.3	13.5	62.9
Cole slaw	122	0.9	3.0	7.5	55.4	12.7	41.7
Potato salad	102	2.7	10.7	2.8	25.0	16.2	64.3
Corn on the cob							
2 to 3 inches	92	2.5	10.9	1.5	14.8	17.0	74.3
4 to 5 inches	169	4.6	10.9	2.8	15.0	31.2	74.1
Kentucky Crisp Fries	156	2.4	6.0	7.5	42.5	20.4	51.4

LONG JOHN SILVER'S SEAFOOD SHOPPES

The peg-legged pirate of *Treasure Island* has lent his seafaring reputation to Long John Silver's, a national chain whose marine motif is reminiscent of the buccaneer's favorite haunt, the Admiral Benbow tavern. The specialty naturally, is fish and shellfish.

Most of the dishes are fried and coated with either batter or breading which puts obstacles in the path of the calorie-conscious. But they can be overcome, because it is possible to order "a la carte," so to speak, buying shrimp ocean scallops, oysters, and other items in portions as small as a single piece (Oysters, incidentally, are a good source of zinc.) By choosing the one-piece rather than the three-piece order of fish with batter, you get only 204 calories a saving of 409. The breaded clams, however, come only in fixed, 5-ounce portions that are among the most calorie-dense (465) dishes on the menu.

Chicken also figures prominently on the menu. Chicken Planks (11! calories per piece) are breasts, and Peg Legs with batter (103 calories per piece' are fried drumsticks. You can mix poultry and piscatorial dishes by ordering the Treasure Chest, which consists of one piece of fish and three Peg Legs (467 calories).

Corn on the cob is a fitting—and filling—accompaniment, well worth the

74 calories. It's a better diet bargain than the quaintly spelled Fryes (as in Frenche Fryes), which come in 3-ounce servings of 275 calories. Another possible choice is the cole slaw; a 4-ounce serving contains 138 calories. Beer and wine are served in some outlets, a touch that the patrons of the Admiral Benbow would have appreciated.

Sauce fanciers should be aware that the dollops can add up. Tartar sauce contains a sobering 75 calories in each tablespoon. A wiser choice is cocktail sauce, which brings only 24 calories with each tablespoon.

This is a suggested day, culminating in dinner at Long John Silver's:

	Calories
BREAKFAST:	
1/2 cup V-8 juice	23
1 1/2 cups Special K cereal with	105
3/4 cup skim milk	66
Coffee or tea	0
	194
LUNCH:	
Danish open-faced sandwich	255
3 ounces sliced turkey	
3 slices tomato	
Lettuce leaves	
1/4 cup alfalfa sprouts	
Mustard	
1 slice pumpernickel bread	
1 large tangerine	46
Iced tea or iced coffee	0
	301
DINNER AT LONG JOHN SILVER'S:	
3 scallops	129
3 shrimp	135
2 oysters	153
1 tablespoon cocktail sauce	24
Corn on the cob	174
Coffee or tea	0
	615
SNACK:	
1 cup skim milk	88

TOTAL CALORIES FOR DAY = 1,198

LONG JOHN SILVER'S SEAFOOD SHOPPES

Item	Calories	Protein		Fat		Carbohydrate	
		grams	% calories	grams	% calories	grams	% calories
Fish with batter							
2-piece order	409	18.8	23.6	18.8	53.1	18.6	23.3
3-piece order	613	28.2	23.6	28.2	53.1	27.9	23.3
Treasure Chest (1 piece fish and 3 Peg Legs)	467	24.6	21.0	28.9	55.6	27.4	23.4
Chicken Planks (4-piece order)	458	27.2	23.8	23.2	45.8	34.7	30.4
Peg Legs with batter (5-piece order)	514	25.3	19.7	32.5	56.9	30.1	23.4
Ocean scallops (6-piece order)	257	10.0	15.6	12.2	42.7	26.8	41.7
Shrimp with batter (6 average order)	269	8.5	12.7	12.5	41.9	30.5	45.4
Breaded oysters (6 pieces)	460	13.5	11.7	19.4	37.9	58.1	50.4
Breaded clams (5 oz.)	465	13.3	11.5	25.2	48.8	46.1	39.7
S.O.S. Super Ocean Sandwich	554	21.6	15.6	30.4	49.2	48.9	35.2
Fryes (3 oz.)	275	3.6	5.2	14.8	48.5	31.8	46.3
Cole slaw (4 oz.)	138	1.0	2.9	8.0	52.0	15.6	45.1
Corn on the cob	174	4.9	11.3	4.3	22.4	28.7	66.3
Hush puppies (3 per order)	153	.9	2.5	6.6	41.0	20.4	56.4
Pecan pie* (3 oz.)	367	4.4	4.8	19.5	47.8	43.6	47.5

*Calculated on the basis of weights provided by Long John Silver's Seafood Shoppes.

McDONALD'S

McDonald's is synonymous with fast food, and the saga of its rise amounts to a modern Horatio Alger tale. The story opens with a humble drive-in in San Bernardino, California, started in 1940 by two brothers named McDonald. The business thrived, attracting the interest of Ray Kroc, a World War I veteran who was then a salesman for milk shake mixing machines. Kroc eventually bought out the brothers and started the chain that today has more than 5,000 outlets and leads the fast food industry in sales. Among children, Ronald McDonald has become a figure almost as well known as Santa Claus. McDonald's even runs its own "university"—known to the alumni as Hamburger U. It teaches subjects ranging from personnel management to french fries.

Frequenters of the Golden Arch have made the Big Mac a legendary lunch. It is to burgers what a double-decker bus is to transportation. The list of ingredients, set to music, is perhaps the world's most famous recipe. We need not repeat them but do need to note that they add up to 541 calories, the high-calorie mark on the McDonald's menu. It's a challenge to the dieter. If you are willing to do without the sauce, you save about 100 calories. And if you removed one of the three bun slices, you would spare yourself about 35. Behold, the Mini Mac.

For those who are able to scale down their ambitions, there is the cheeseburger, which harbors a relatively modest 306 calories, fewer even than the Filet-O-Fish (402). The Egg McMuffin has convinced many non-breakfast eaters to change their habits, even though it starts off the morning with 352 calories.

A good reason to go easy on the "entree" is that many people find the french fries among the most tempting items. At only 211 calories (small order), it's worth giving in to temptation and going easier on calories at another meal.

A tip for shake lovers: Ordering vanilla instead of chocolate will save you 41 calories (323 versus 364). A glass of plain milk, of course, would cut the calories in half (160).

Below is a suggestion for planning your day around a dinner at McDonald's. Since the dinner is low in vitamin A, the lunch includes carrots and apricots. Together they easily fulfill the daily requirements for that vitamin (NDS = more than 4,000).

	Calories
BREAKFAST:	
1 sliced small banana with	85
1 cup 100% Bran Flakes and	150
3/4 cup skim milk	66
Coffee or tea	0
	301
LUNCH:	
Chef's salad:	210
1 ounce julienne strips turkey	
1 ounce julienne strips Swiss cheese	

	Calories
1/4 cup alfalfa sprouts	
1/2 sliced medium cucumber (unpeeled)	
1 cup shredded lettuce	
1 sliced medium tomato	
1/2 grated carrot	
2 tablespoons low-calorie dressing	30
6 Wheat Thins	54
4 apricot halves (water-packed)	50
	344

DINNER AT McDONALD'S:

1 cheeseburger	306
1 small french fries	211
1 tablespoon ketchup	18
Coffee	0
	535

TOTAL CALORIES FOR DAY = 1,180

McDONALD'S

Item	Calories	Protein		Fat		Carbohydrate	
		grams	% calories	grams	% calories	grams	% calorie
Egg McMuffin	352	18.0	20.0	19.6	50.0	26.0	30.0
Hot cakes with butter and syrup	472	8.0	6.8	9.3	17.7	88.9	75.5
Scrambled eggs	162	11.6	28.8	11.9	66.5	1.9	4.7
Hash brown potatoes	130	1.3	3.9	8.1	54.7	13.8	41.4
Pork sausage	184	8.6	18.7	16.6	81.2	0.1	-
English muffin (buttered)	186	5.6	12.0	5.6	27.1	28.3	60.9
Hamburger	257	12.9	20.1	9.4	32.9	30.2	47.0
Cheeseburger	306	15.6	20.4	13.4	39.4	30.8	40.2
Quarter-Pounder	418	25.6	24.5	20.5	44.1	32.9	31.4
Quarter-Pounder with cheese	518	30.9	23.9	28.6	49.7	34.2	26.4
Big Mac	541	25.6	18.9	31.4	52.2	39.0	28.8

		McDONALD'S (continued)					
Item	Calories	Protein		Fat		Carbohydrate	
		grams	% calories	grams	% calories	grams	% calories
Filet-O-Fish	402	15.1	15.0	22.7	50.8	34.3	34.1
French fries							
Small	211	3.1	5.9	10.6	45.2	25.8	48.9
Large	362	5.3	5.9	18.2	45.2	44.3	48.9
Chocolate shake	364	10.7	11.8	9.0	22.3	59.8	65.9
Vanilla shake	323	10.1	12.5	8.4	23.4	51.7	64.0
Strawberry shake	345	10.2	11.8	8.5	22.1	57.3	66.2
Apple pie	300	2.2	2.9	18.6	55.8	31.0	41.3
Cherry pie	298	2.2	3.0	17.6	53.3	32.5	43.8
McDonald-land Cookies	294	4.3	5.9	10.6	32.4	45.4	61.8
Sundaes							
Hot fudge	290	6.2	8.5	9.8	30.3	44.6	61.2
Caramel	282	4.9	6.9	6.6	21.1	50.8	72.0
Strawberry	229	4.2	7.3	4.0	15.7	44.1	77.0
Pineapple	230	4.2	7.3	4.6	18.0	42.9	74.7

ORANGE JULIUS

It could have been called the Orange Irving. Or the Orange Sidney. But it so happened that the Los Angeles store manager who first sold the drink in 1926 was named Julius. The customers kept coming in to order "An Orange, Julius." And the name stuck.

When Julius was in charge of the mixing, it was considered a health drink. Although no longer viewed as an elixir, the sweet, frothy concoction has a large band of devotees.

The Orange Julius is marketed today by a California-based chain that has 520 outlets in the United States and other countries. The outlets offer a variety of burger and hot dog dishes, but the big attraction is the famous beverage.

Although the formula is a closely guarded trade secret, the calorie count is known: 149 for a 12-ounce glass. That compares favorably with the same amount of milk (240 calories) and plain orange juice (180), the first cousin of the Julius. Twelve ounces of soda would be only one calorie more, but the thickness of the Julius makes it a much more sensual experience, an important consideration for the dieter who feels deprived.

There is even a nutritional bonus. The Julius is relatively high in vitamin C. It supplies about two-thirds of your daily requirements for that nutrient achieving a Nutrient Density Score of more than 1,000.

The Orange Julius has spawned other fruit drinks: the Pineapple Julius and Strawberry, Banana, Peach, and Lemon versions. Purists were skeptical at first, but few wished to stand in the path of progress.

The following is a meal plan that will allow you to sample one of these drinks:

	Calories
BREAKFAST:	
3/4 cup oatmeal with	98
3 chopped dates and	66
3/4 cup skim milk	66
Coffee or tea	0
	230
LUNCH:	
Ham salad:	159
2 ounces diced ham	
2 tablespoons cottage cheese	
1 diced celery stalk	
1/8 teaspoon dried mustard	
1/8 teaspoon prepared horseradish	
Lettuce leaf	
1 slice pumpernickel bread	79
1 cup skim milk	88
	326
TREAT AT ORANGE JULIUS:	
1 small Orange Julius (12 ounces)	149
DINNER:	
Oriental chicken:	357
3 ounces diced cooked chicken	
3 ounces snow peas	
5 leaves of Swiss chard or spinach	
1/2 cup sliced mushrooms (fresh)	
1/2 cup bean sprouts	

	Calories
cook in preheated saucepan until vegetables are wilted; add 2 tablespoons soy sauce; garnish with 1 tablespoon slivered almonds	
1/3 cup cooked rice	74
1 small apple	58
Coffee or tea	0
	489

TOTAL CALORIES FOR DAY = 1,194

ORANGE JULIUS

Item	Calories	Protein		Fat		Carbohydrate	
		grams	% calories	grams	% calories	grams	% calories
Orange Julius (small, 12 oz.)	149	1.2	3.2	0.4	2.1	36.0	94.7

PIZZA HUT

A hallowed date in the annals of Pizza Hut is August 6, 1958—the day the original restaurant, in Wichita, Kansas, placed its first 100-pound order for mozzarella. Less than 20 years later it was ordering cheese in million-pound units, and the chain, an outgrowth of a family grocery store, was giving corporate competition to mom-and-pop pizzerias throughout the country. Today its ovens are feeding Italian-style appetites in such unlikely places as Kuwait.

The red and white tablecloths follow traditional decor, but Pizza Hut has made a breakthrough by inventing a heat-retaining carry-out carton (for a few cents extra) that enables you to enjoy warm pizza at home without exceeding the 55-mile-an-hour speed limit.

Eating at the restaurant also may be a more relaxed experience, when you compare the pace with that of most fast food outlets. A full-dress pizza requires 15 to 20 minutes of baking time.

You can use this time to fill a bowl at the salad bar. That will give you additional vitamin C, which is needed because no respectable pizza would be baked at less than 500 degrees, destroying most of the C. The salad also takes the edge off your hunger so that you can more easily limit your meal to two slices or modest helpings of the pasta dishes that are also on the menu. More-over, strolling between the table and the salad bar provides exercise.

A word of advice: Since the salad bar does not have low-calorie dressing, use vinegar. Similarly, pass up the free peppermint candies; they may not cost you extra money but they do cost extra calories. You should also realize that every 12 ounces of the beer contains 150 calories and not many nutrients, except for chromium.

The lowest-calorie pizza is the Thin'n Crispy cheese version. But the Thick'n Chewy version is worth the extra 50 calories. It has been selected (with extra cheese) for this day's diet plan:

	Calories
BREAKFAST:	
1/2 cup unsweetened grapefruit juice	44
1 cup 100% Bran Flakes with	150
3/4 cup skim milk and	66
1/2 sliced small banana	43
Coffee or tea	0
	303
LUNCH:	
Salmon plate:	220
3 ounces pink salmon (canned)	
6 asparagus spears	
1 sliced medium tomato	
1/2 sliced medium cucumber (unpeeled)	
1 slice Bermuda onion	
Lettuce leaves	
Lemon wedges	
6 Wheat Thins	54
1 large tangerine	46
Coffee or tea	0
	320
DINNER AT PIZZA HUT:	
2 slices Thick'n Chewy Super Style cheese pizza	450
(from a 13-inch pizza)	
1 serving from salad bar:	115
1 cup lettuce	
1/4 cup cucumber	
1/4 cup sprouts	
1/4 cup celery	

	Calories
1/4 cup beans	
2 tablespoons beets	
1 tablespoon Bac-O Bits	
Vinegar or lemon	
Iced tea	0
	565

TOTAL CALORIES FOR DAY = 1,188

PIZZA HUT*

Item	Calories	Protein		Fat		Carbohydrate	
		grams	% calories	grams	% calories	grams	% calories
(2 slices of medium pizza)							
THIN'N CRISPY® pizza:							
Standard cheese	340	19	22.1	11	28.9	42	49.0
Super Style cheese	410	26	25.4	14	30.7	45	43.9
Standard pepperoni	370	19	20.1	15	35.6	42	44.3
Super Style pepperoni	430	23	21.2	19	39.3	43	39.5
Standard pork/ mushroom	380	21	21.8	14	32.6	44	45.6
Super Style pork/ mushroom	450	26	22.7	19	37.2	46	40.1
Supreme	400	21	20.3	17	37.1	44	42.6
Super supreme	520	30	22.3	26	43.5	46	34.2
THICK'N CHEWY® pizza:							
Standard cheese	390	24	24.1	10	22.6	53	53.3
Super Style cheese	450	31	26.6	14	27.0	54	46.4
Standard pepperoni	450	25	22.1	16	31.9	52	46.0

*PIZZA HUT, THICK'N CHEWY and THIN'N CRISPY are trademarks of PIZZA HUT, INC.

PIZZA HUT (continued

Item	Calories	Protein		Fat		Carbohydrate	
		grams	% calories	grams	% calories	grams	% calories
Super Style pepperoni	490	27	21.8	20	36.3	52	41.9
Standard pork/ mushroom	430	27	24.2	14	28.3	53	47.5
Super Style pork/ mushroom	500	30	24.1	18	32.5	54	43.4
Supreme	480	29	23.9	18	33.3	52	42.8
Super supreme	590	34	23.0	26	39.7	55	37.3

RUSTLER STEAK HOUSE

From a distance you pick out the silhouette of a cowboy town. But this is up-state New York, not Old Tucson, you say, and you pull into the parking lot for a closer look. It is a Rustler Steak House, decorated with mementos from the gunslinging era. These days, however, they are slinging mainly steaks, sea-food, and sandwiches in a cafeteria-style, family restaurant atmosphere.

Despite its Western motif, the 150-unit Rustler chain started by selling T-bones to tenderfoots. The outlets were concentrated in the mid-Atlantic states before 1973, when the chain began to spread to other parts of the country.

Whatever its origin, the Wild West theme is firmly fixed and is even carried out by the extensive salad bar. It's called a "salad corral," and you can lasso a wide variety of low-calorie ingredients, including bean sprouts, green beans, and cherry tomatoes. That provides a good opportunity for the dieter to fill up at relatively small caloric cost and also get some fiber. Go easy on the dressing, through. (The salad bar is identical to the one at Gino's, a related chain.)

Among the main dishes, the seafood combination platter is the highest in calories (1,167); it combines clams, shrimp, and a cod fillet. Close behind is the cod fish platter (1,147). In all the platters, a substantial proportion of the calories (268) comes from the margarine on the baked potato and roll. You can easily spare yourself those extra calories by asking for the potato and roll without the margarine.

This is how to sashay into Rustler without exceeding your daily calorie quota:

	Calories
BREAKFAST:	
1/2 cup stewed prunes (unsweetened)	127
2/3 cup Wheat Chex cereal with	110
1/2 cup skimmed milk	44
Coffee or tea	0
	281
LUNCH:	
Fruit delight:	
1 cup low-fat, plain yogurt (or 1/2 cup low-fat cottage cheese)	130
1/2 cup fresh or frozen blueberries (or 3/4 cup strawberries)	45
1 sliced small orange	49
1/2 sliced small banana	43
3 saltine crackers	36
Coffee or tea	0
	303
DINNER AT RUSTLER STEAK HOUSE:	
Rib-eye steak platter (normally 765 calories, but order it without margarine on the roll and potato)	497
1 serving of salad from salad bar:	75
take a lot of lettuce and a variety of other ingredients; go easy on the cheese, Bac-O Bits, and chick peas; instead of dressing use lemon juice and pepper	
Coffee or tea	0
	572

TOTAL CALORIES FOR DAY = 1,156

RUSTLER STEAK HOUSE

Item	Calories	Protein		Fat		Carbohydrate	
		grams	% calories	grams	% calories	grams	% calories
Platters							
(all with potato with margarine, roll with margarine):							
Beef patty							
4 oz.	804	27.5	14.1	49.0	56.3	58.0	29.6
7 oz.	1,001	42.1	17.4	63.0	58.6	58.0	24.0
Rib-eye steak	765	27.7	14.5	46.7	55.1	58.0	30.4
Rustler (strip steak)	878	41.3	18.9	53.1	54.6	58.0	26.5
Filet mignon	849	42.7	20.2	49.1	52.3	58.0	27.5
T-bone steak	899	48.4	22.2	52.1	52.4	58.0	25.9
Steak and crab	1,020	38.6	15.1	70.3	62.0	58.4	22.9
Clam	945	22.4	9.5	59.7	56.9	79.2	33.6
Shrimp	926	35.4	15.4	49.9	48.8	82.3	35.8
Cod	1,147	43.5	15.1	73.4	57.3	79.4	27.7
Seafood combination	1,167	43.1	14.8	72.4	55.8	86.0	29.4
SANDWICHES:							
Trailboss	553	33.6	25.5	29.5	50.3	32.0	24.2
Westerner	467	24.4	21.6	19.6	39.0	44.6	39.4
Steak	369	22.0	23.6	16.6	40.1	33.7	36.2
SANDWICH ACCESSORIES:							
Potato chips	82	0.8	3.9	5.6	61.5	7.1	34.6
Cheese (2 slices)	92	5.8	25.4	7.4	72.9	0.4	1.7
Potato (with 2 tbs.	155	4.3	10.7	0.2	1.1	35.3	88.1
margarine)	215	0.2	0.4	23.0	99.3	0.1	0.2
Roll	117	3.5	12.0	1.4	10.8	22.6	77.3
Jello (cherry)	75	1.5	7.4	0.1	1.1	18.6	91.5
Pudding (chocolate)	144	3.4	9.1	2.8	16.8	27.7	74.1
Pie (1/6 of pie)*							
Apple	410	3.4	3.3	17.8	38.3	61.0	58.4
Blueberry	387	3.8	3.8	17.3	39.4	56.0	56.7
Custard	327	9.2	11.3	16.6	45.7	35.1	43.0
Lemon meringue	357	5.2	5.8	14.3	35.7	52.8	58.6

RUSTLER STEAK HOUSE (continued)

Item	Calories	Protein		Fat		Carbohydrate	
		grams	% calories	grams	% calories	grams	% calories
Salad bar items:							
Lettuce (2 oz.)	7	0.5	23.8	-	-	1.6	76.2
Onions (1 oz.)	11	0.4	13.8	-	-	2.5	86.2
Tomato (2 oz.)	13	0.6	17.0	0.1	6.4	2.7	76.6
Cucumbers (½ oz.)	2	0.1	16.7	-	-	0.5	83.3
Radishes (¾ oz.)	4	0.2	20.0	-	-	0.8	80.0
Celery (½ oz.)	2	0.1	14.3	-	-	0.6	85.7
Carrots (¼ oz.)	3	0.1	12.5	-	-	0.7	87.5
Kidney beans (1 oz.)	26	1.6	24.9	0.1	3.5	4.6	71.6
Chick peas (1 oz.)	102	5.8	22.1	1.4	12.0	17.3	65.9
Beets (1 oz.)	10	0.3	10.7	-	-	2.5	89.3
Green beans (1 oz.)	7	0.4	18.8	0.1	10.6	1.5	70.6
Peperoncini (½ oz.)	5	0.2	13.3	-	-	1.3	86.7
Bean sprouts (1 oz.)	8	0.9	34.3	0.1	8.6	1.5	57.1
Bac-O Bits (¼ oz.)	29	2.8	38.4	1.2	37.0	1.8	24.6
Grated cheese food (¼ oz.)	28	2.6	38.0	1.8	59.1	0.2	2.9
Green peppers (¾ oz.)	5	0.2	16.7	-	-	1.0	83.3
Dressings (1 tbs.)							
Italian	60	-	-	7.0	94.0	1.0	6.0
French	60	-	-	6.0	87.1	2.0	12.9
Russian	60	-	-	6.0	87.1	2.0	12.9
Bleu cheese	80	1.0	5.3	8.0	94.7	-	-

*Calculated on the basis of serving sizes provided by Rustler Steak House.

TACO BELL

Its prize dishes are not quite as American as apple pie, but since its founding in southern California in 1962, the Taco Bell chain has won converts to Mexican-style food in 40 states and Guam. Although there is no mariachi band, the menu makes you think you are south of the border—except that the octane level has been lowered for the north-of-the-border palate. The staple and namesake dish is the taco, a crisp corn tortilla (pancake) filled with ground beef, sauce, lettuce, and shredded cheddar cheese. Other dishes elaborate upon the basic tortilla, resulting in a variety of interesting shapes, colors, and textures. All are surprising calorie bargains.

Despite its panoply of ingredients—sour cream, lettuce, tomatoes, cheese, olives, pinto beans, and ground beef—the Beefy Tostada has only 291 calories. There is also a nutritional bonus: The dish achieves a relatively high Nutrient Density Score for a number of vitamins and minerals. The following are all above 100: protein (270), vitamin A (563), thiamin (104), riboflavin (147), niacin (166), vitamin C (138), calcium (170), and iron (123). The tostada even rates as a low-sodium dish (only 138 mg). Here is how to work one into your day:

	Calories
BREAKFAST:	
1 slice small banana with	85
1 cup plain, low-fat yogurt and dash of cinnamon	150
1 slice whole wheat toast with	65
1/2 teaspoon margarine	17
Coffee or tea	0
	317
LUNCH AT TACO BELL:	
Beefy tostada	291
Iced tea with lemon	0
	291
DINNER:	
1 cup chicken bouillon with dill	8
6 ounces broiled flank steak	300
1 small (5 ounce) baked potato with	106
1 tablespoon sour cream	30
6 asparagus spears	26
1 cup mixed salad greens with	20
2 tablespoons low-calorie salad dressing	30
1/2 fresh grapefruit	55
Coffee or tea	0
	575

TOTAL CALORIES FOR DAY = 1,183

TACO BELL

Item	Calories	Protein		Fat		Carbohydrate	
		grams	% calories	grams	% calories	grams	% calories
Taco	159	10.4	26.0	9.1	51.4	9.2	22.6
Pintos 'n' Cheese	231	12.3	19.7	11.3	40.8	24.6	39.5
Tostada	206	15.1	29.3	9.2	40.2	15.8	30.5
Bean burrito	345	13.6	15.8	11.1	28.8	47.9	55.4
Enchirito	391	23.3	23.8	20.9	48.1	27.5	28.1
Beefy tostada	291	17.8	24.1	14.9	45.4	22.6	30.5
Bellbeefer	243	13.5	22.3	8.2	30.3	28.9	47.4
Burrito Supreme	387	17.8	19.0	16.9	40.4	38.1	40.6

TACO CHARLEY

Taco Charley, named for a founding executive, is another missionary for Mexican cooking. Within four years of its opening in 1975, the chain had 30 outlets and a blueprint for expansion from California and Nevada into Arizona.

Taco Charley offers the customary varieties of taco, burrito, enchilada, and tostada, but it also compromises with standard American tastes by selling a hybrid called Taco-in-a-Bun (alias The Charley). It has the familiar feel of a burger in the hand but between the layers of bread are stuffed taco fillings.

Those who miss the chewy, corny taste of the tortilla would be better off, especially calorically, trying the conventional taco. In the soft form, it is only 200 calories. Exercising your option for the crispy taco will not cost you any extra calories. If crispness is your fancy, you would probably like tortilla chips. They are only 170 calories, but the serving (1.27 oz.) could hardly be other than a snack. Nachos, tortilla chips holding mounds of beans, cheese sauce, and other ingredients, are equally tempting, but the caloric grand total is more than 700.

It is possible to put together vegetarian meals around, for example, the tosta grande or the bean burrito. Like the beef and combination styles, the bean burrito comes in both hot and mild versions, depending on your choice of sauce. Neither version is really incendiary, but the choice can affect the calorie levels slightly. For a few pennies more, extra tomatoes (a dieting plus) or extra sour cream (a dieting minus) are added to any entree.

Below is a typical day with a stop at Taco Charley. The tosta grande provides iron, vitamin A, riboflavin, and niacin. The extra tomatoes on the taco boost the day's vitamin C total.

	Calories
BREAKFAST:	
3/4 cup orange juice	90
1 poached egg on	88
1 slice whole wheat toast	65
Coffee or tea	0
	243
LUNCH:	
1 cup low-fat cottage cheese with	120
4 apricot halves (water-packed) and	50
2 tablespoons slivered almonds	86
1 cup shredded lettuce	8
6 Wheat Thins	54
Coffee or tea	0
	318
DINNER AT TACO CHARLEY:	
Crisp taco (comes with beef, lettuce, cheese; ask for tomatoes—10 calories extra)	210
Tosta grande (comes with frijoles or beans, cheese, tomatoes, olives, sour cream)	300
Jalapeño pepper (optional)	(4)
Iced tea	0
	510 (514)
SNACK:	
Late-night crunchies:	30
1/2 cup raw cauliflower	
1 small raw green pepper, cut into strips	
1 cup skim milk	88
	118

TOTAL CALORIES FOR DAY = 1,189 (1,193)

TACO CHARLEY

Item	Calories	Protein		Fat		Carbohydrate	
		grams	% calories	grams	% calories	grams	% calories
Soft taco	200	10	20.7	13	60.6	9	18.7
Crisp taco	200	10	20.3	13	59.4	10	20.3
Burrito grande	460	19	16.7	19	37.6	52	45.7

TACO CHARLEY (continued)

Item	Calories	Protein		Fat		Carbohydrate	
		grams	% calories	grams	% calories	grams	% calories
Beef burrito							
spicy sauce	430	22	20.4	19	39.7	43	39.9
mild sauce	430	21	19.6	20	42.1	41	38.3
Bean burrito							
spicy sauce	360	13	14.3	11	27.3	53	58.4
mild sauce	370	13	14.0	11	26.7	55	59.3
Combination burrito							
spicy sauce	420	18	17.1	16	34.3	51	48.6
mild sauce	415	18	17.5	15	32.9	51	49.6
Enchilada	350	16	18.6	17	44.3	32	37.1
Tosta grande	300	15	19.7	16	47.4	25	32.9
Tostada	200	8	16.0	8	36.0	24	48.0
Charley (Taco-in-a-Bun)	280	14	19.8	11	35.0	32	45.2
Frijoles (6.6 oz.)	250	12	18.6	10	34.9	30	46.5
Tortilla chips (1.27 oz.)	170	3	6.8	8	40.9	23	52.3

WENDY'S OLD FASHIONED HAMBURGERS

Wendy's serves the burger equivalent of the Hanging Gardens of Babylon. It's the triple hamburger with cheese, constructed of three-quarters of a pound of meat and landscaped with lettuce, tomato, onions, pickles, relish, mayonnaise, ketchup, and mustard. That Gargantuan creation typifies the menu at Wendy's, which was founded in 1969 by R. David Thomas and named for his daughter. The more than 1,700 outlets concentrate on burgers—and on making them big.

The smallest of Wendy's "hot 'n' juicy" specialities is the quater-pound single hamburger (472 calories). Three meat patties of that size go into the triple with cheese. (The patties, incidentally, are made square, so that you can see the corners sticking out from under the bun.) The triple easily overfulfills your protein requirement for the day (165 percent of the RDA), but it also packs 1,036 calories, virtually the entire daily quota for the dieter. It would also be a rather high-fat day, drawing almost 59 percent of its calories from that nutrient.

Fortunately for the dieter, every burger can be ordered with the same fixings as the triple, so even the single burger can be festive, although it may lack the drama of the multi-layered version. Saying "hold the mayo" will save you at least 50 calories, bringing the single down to 422.

Cooked burgers that are not sold within a few minutes are recycled into chili, the only nonburger main dish. The chili is high in cayenne pepper but relatively low in garlic and calories (229).

Here is a day with lunch at Wendy's:

	Calories
BREAKFAST:	
3/4 cup tomato juice	35
1 cup Total cereal with	108
1 cup skim milk	88
Coffee or tea	0
	231
LUNCH AT WENDY'S:	
Single hamburger (without mayonnaise)	422
Iced tea with lemon	0
	422
DINNER:	
Pasta with clam sauce:	245
heat contents of a 7 1/2-ounce can of minced clams with parsley and garlic; serve on 2/3 cup cooked enriched spaghetti with 1 tablespoon grated parmesan cheese	
Spinach salad:	34
1 cup spinach	
1 sliced small tomato	
4 sliced large mushrooms (fresh)	
1 tablespoon low-calorie French dressing	15
2/3 cup steamed Italian green beans	46
Espresso with a twist of lemon, or coffee or tea	0
1/2 cup fresh or frozen raspberries (unsweetened)	51
	391
SNACK:	
Blueberry banana treat:	155
Mix in a blender or food processor	
1 cup skim milk	
1/2 cup frozen blueberries (unsweetened)	
1/2 small banana	
Dash of cinnamon	

TOTAL CALORIES FOR DAY = 1,199

WENDY'S OLD FASHIONED HAMBURGERS

Item	Calories	Protein grams	Protein % calories	Fat grams	Fat % calories	Carbohydrate grams	Carbohydrate % calories
Hamburgers							
Single	472	25.7	21.8	26.1	49.7	33.6	28.5
Double	669	44.1	26.3	39.6	53.3	34.0	20.4
Triple	853	64.5	30.3	51.4	54.2	33.1	15.5
Single with cheese	577	32.6	22.6	34.5	53.8	34.1	23.6
Double with cheese	797	49.8	25.0	48.2	54.5	40.9	20.5
Triple with cheese	1,036	71.6	27.7	67.7	58.8	35.0	13.5
Chili	229	19.5	34.1	7.6	29.8	20.6	36.1
French fries	327	5.1	6.3	15.9	43.6	41.0	50.1
Frosty	391	8.6	8.7	15.9	36.6	53.6	54.7

NOTE: Because Wendy's hamburgers are prepared according to each customer's order, significant variations in the test results will occur. The values provide only a general guideline.

WHITE CASTLE

White Castle can plausibly claim to have pioneered in the fast food business, but today it seems—proudly—in the industry's rearguard. Its conservatism expresses itself in such old-fashioned notions as avoiding growth. The White Castle chain has added fewer than 150 outlets since it opened its first turreted restaurant in Wichita, Kansas, in 1921. (The architecture was borrowed from another Midwestern monument, Chicago's Water Tower.) It retains its hospital-like, all-white decor, a stylistic innovation that has had few imitators.

The burgers still sell at almost Depression-era prices, partly because they are kept relatively small (.75 ounces per patty). The chain maintains it was the first to squash down the original meatball-shaped burger for ease of cooking. The burgers were also made square to fit more efficiently on a grill (an unexpected boon for the energy crisis) and punched with five holes, like dominoes, so they can be steam-cooked over onions without being turned.

The menu is pristinely limited. In general, if you are not in a White Castle for a burger, you are in the wrong place. The chain urges you to "take home a sackful," but a dieter's compromise would be to down a double cheeseburger (305 calories), composed of two of White Castle's standard-gauge patties and cheese. That saves one bun and 65 calories. Skip the shoestring french fries and content yourself with iced tea. For an even lighter meal, you can try the fish sandwich at 192 calories, perhaps adding cheese for only 25 extra calories and a dash of tartar sauce for 25 more.

A plan for a day's eating with a White Castle lunch follows. The rest of the meals provide balance by offering vitamin A, iron, calcium, vitamin C, and folacin. Just the spinach at dinner contains 410 percent of the RDA for vitamin A, almost 30 percent for iron, 30 percent for calcium, 50 percent for vitamin C, and 40 percent for folacin.

	Calories
BREAKFAST:	
1/2 fresh grapefruit	55
1 poached egg on	88
1/2 toasted English muffin	70
Coffee or tea	0
	213
LUNCH AT WHITE CASTLE:	
1 double cheeseburger	305
Iced tea	0
	305
DINNER:	
4 ounces broiled veal with lemon and garlic	186
1 small (5-ounce) baked potato with	106
1 teaspoon margarine	34
1 cup spinach, dash of nutmeg, black pepper	53
1 cup salad greens	20
1 cup skim milk	88
Coffee or tea	0
3/4 cup fresh pineapple (or 1 large slice canned pineapple, packed in juice)	55
	542
SNACK:	
Late-night crunchies:	46
1 small carrot	
1 large celery stalk	
1 small green pepper	
1 cup skim milk	88
	134

TOTAL CALORIES FOR DAY = 1,194

WHITE CASTLE

Item	Calories	Protein		Fat		Carbohydrate	
		grams	% calories	grams	% calories	grams	% calories
French fries (2.6 oz.)	225	3.1	5.6	10.8	44.3	27.4	50.1
Hamburger	160	6.0	15.5	6.8	39.5	17.5	45.0
Double hamburger	255	9.8	15.8	13.1	47.6	22.6	36.6
Cheeseburger	185	7.8	17.3	8.7	43.6	17.6	39.1
Double cheeseburger	305	13.4	18.0	16.9	51.2	22.9	30.8
Fish sandwich (without tartar sauce)	192	7.4	15.7	8.5	41.0	20.2	43.3
Double fish sandwich	319	12.5	16.1	16.5	47.8	28.0	36.1
Fish sandwich with cheese	217	9.2	17.4	10.4	44.2	20.3	38.4
Double fish sandwich with cheese	369	16.2	18.0	20.2	50.6	28.2	30.6

WIENERSCHNITZEL

Wienerschnitzel began in 1961 as "Der Wienerschnitzel," a basic hot dog and french fries operation in Wilmington, California. Along the way, it subtracted the "der" and added burgers. Today it has more than 300 outlets, concentrated in California and the Southwest and catering heavily to the drive-through trade.

Wienerschnitzel's name might lead you to expect menu items like sauerbraten-on-a-bun. Actually, there is nothing more Teutonic than a Kraut Dog, the standard American hot dog with sauerkraut, an East Coast specialty moved West.

There *is* something Polish, though, at least in theory. It's the Polish Sandwich, a combination of sausage, melted Swiss cheese, sauerkraut, pickle, and mustard on rye (404 calories).

The Super Deluxe amalgamates a quarter-pound burger patty, lettuce, pickle, ketchup, mustard, sliced onion, and a mayonnaise-type sauce. If you get it without the sauce, you save about 75 calories, bringing the total down to

397. Tomato, cheese, and chili topping are also available for an extra charge—and, for the last two, about 40 extra calories each.

Either the Polish Sandwich or the Super Deluxe is probably a better diet choice than the Corn Dog, a hot dog enveloped in deep-fried corn meal batter. The Corn Dog provides a change for those who are bored by buns (you eat it on a stick), but it uses quite a few calories (520) to make a relatively modest dent in your appetite.

Dieters should also be aware that when Wienerschnitzel's menu says "large," it really means it. The large soft drinks are a full quart (about 350 calories, allowing for ice), and the large order of french fries weighs about half a pound (687 calories). Stick to the smaller portions or share with several friends.

There are some diet pluses. The iced tea is not presweetened, and salad bars have begun to appear in Wienerschnitzel outlets.

What follows is a day that includes lunch at Wienerschnitzel and a snack. The broccoli at dinner helps balance the day nutritionally by adding vitamins A and C, iron, and fiber.

	Calories
BREAKFAST:	
3/4 cup tomato juice	35
1 cup Total cereal with	108
3/4 cup skim milk	66
Coffee or tea	0
	209
LUNCH AT WIENERSCHNITZEL:	
Polish Sandwich	404
Iced tea	0
	404
DINNER:	
1 cup chicken bouillon with minced parsley	8
1/2 baked or broiled chicken breast:	228
marinate and baste with 1 tablespoon corn oil,	
2 tablespoons lemon juice, garlic, thyme,	
pepper, 1/2 tablespoon finely chopped onion	
1 cup broccoli	40
1 small (5-ounce) baked potato with dill	106
1 cup mixed salad greens with	20
2 tablespoons low-calorie salad dressing	30

	Calories
1 small apple	58
Coffee or tea	0
	490

SNACK:

1 cup skim milk	88

TOTAL CALORIES FOR DAY = 1,191

WIENERSCHNITZEL

Item	Calories	Protein		Fat		Carbohydrate	
		grams	% calories	grams	% calories	grams	% calories
Super Deluxe	472	25.7	21.8	26.1	49.7	33.6	28.5
Corn Dog	520	11.1	8.5	28.9	50.0	53.9	41.5
Polish Sandwich	404	21.0	21.3	27.8	63.4	15.1	15.3
Kraut Dog	241	8.4	14.0	13.0	48.7	22.4	37.3
Chili Dog	269	9.2	14.1	14.3	49.2	24.0	36.7
Chili-Cheese Dog	311	13.3	16.7	18.6	52.5	24.6	30.8
French fries*							
2.5 oz.	215	3.0	5.7	10.7	45.7	25.6	48.6
4 oz.	343	4.8	5.7	17.7	45.7	41.0	48.6
8 oz.	687	9.6	5.7	35.3	45.7	82.0	48.6
Hot apple pie* (4 oz.)	350	3.3	3.8	19.7	50.6	40.0	45.6

*Calculated on the basis of weights provided by Wienerschnitzel.

APPENDIX A:
Condiments, Drinks, and
Salad Bar Ingredients

The typical fast food meal is accompanied by a variety of condiments and drinks, and sometimes a do-it-yourself salad bar is at hand. The following tables list the calories of the items you are most likely to encounter.

CONDIMENTS

Item (1 tablespoon unless otherwise noted)	Calories
A-1 Sauce	13
Butter	102
Cheese (1 slice)	40-100
Cocktail sauce	24
Horseradish dressing	55
Jalapeño pepper	4
Ketchup	18
Margarine	102
Mayonnaise	100
Mustard	12
Onion	4
Pickle, dill (3 slices or 1 spear)	2
Pickle relish	20
Sauerkraut (¼ cup)	10
Sour cream	26
Soy sauce	6
Sugar	40
Taco sauce	4
Tartar sauce	75
Tomato slice	3
Worcestershire sauce	10

DRINKS

Item	Amount	Calories
Beer	12 oz.	155
Chocolate, hot	6 oz.	206
Coffee		0
Cola	10 oz.	129
Diet soda	16 oz.	1
Dr. Pepper	10 oz.	122
Ginger ale	10 oz.	106
Half and half	1 tbs.	20
Milk	8 oz.	144-170
Milk, chocolate	8 oz.	210
Nondairy creamer, dry	1 tsp.	12
Nondairy creamer, liquid	1 tbs.	25
Orange drink	8 oz.	84-122
Orange juice	8 oz.	93-129
Root beer	10 oz.	137
Shake, vanilla	small	310-391
Tea		0
Tomato juice	8 oz.	47
Water		0
Wine, red	4 oz.	85
Wine, white	4 oz.	86

SALAD BAR INGREDIENTS

Item	Amount	Calories
Alfalfa sprouts	½ cup	11
Bacon bits (imitation)	1 tbs.	24
Bean sprouts	2 tbs.	5
Beets	2 tbs. (cooked, sliced)	7
Carrots	2 tbs. (shredded)	6
Celery	2 tbs. (chopped)	3
Cheese, American	1 tbs. (shredded)	26
Cheese, parmesan	1 tbs. (grated)	21
Cottage cheese	¼ cup	58
Chick peas	2 tbs. (cooked)	40
Croutons	2 tbs.	18
Cucumbers	¼ cup (diced)	5
Eggs, hard-boiled	1 tbs. (chopped)	14
Green beans	2 tbs. (cooked, sliced)	4
Green peppers	¼ cup (sliced)	5
Kidney beans	2 tbs. (cooked)	27
Lettuce	1 cup (shredded)	8
Radishes	4 medium	3

SALAD BAR INGREDIENTS (continued)

Item	Amount	Calories
Tomato	1 medium	33
Tomato, cherry	4 whole	12
Dressings		
Blue cheese	2 tbs.	114-160
French	2 tbs.	106-156
Italian	2 tbs.	124-174
Lemon juice	2 tbs.	8
Low-calorie dressings	2 tbs.	15-30
Oil	2 tbs.	250
Russian or thousand island	2 tbs.	118-156
Vinegar	2 tbs.	6

APPENDIX B:
The One-Week Fast Food Diet Plan

The menus on the preceding pages demonstrate how to plan a reasonably balanced diet day that includes a fast food meal. This section presents a plan for a whole week of healthful dieting with two full meals and a snack at a fast food restaurant—a typical American eating pattern. The levels of nutrients vary somewhat from day to day, but the weekly averages are adequate. Best of all, by following the plan, you should be able to lose up to 3 pounds for the week.

DAY 1

	Calories
BREAKFAST:	
1 sliced small banana with	85
1 cup 100% Bran Flakes and	150
3/4 cup skim milk	66
Coffee or tea	0
	301
LUNCH:	
Chef's salad:	210
1 ounce julienne strips turkey	
1 ounce julienne strips Swiss cheese	
1/4 cup alfalfa sprouts	
1/2 sliced medium cucumber (unpeeled)	
1 cup shredded lettuce	
1 sliced medium tomato	

	Calories
1/2 grated carrot	
2 tablespoons low-calorie dressing	30
6 Wheat Thins	54
4 apricot halves (water-packed)	50
	344

DINNER AT McDONALD'S:

1 cheeseburger	306
1 small french fries	211
1 tablespoon ketchup	18
Coffee	0
	535

TOTAL CALORIES FOR DAY = 1,180

DAY 2

	Calories

BREAKFAST:

1/2 medium grapefruit	55
1 poached egg	88
1 slice whole wheat toast	65
Coffee or tea	0
	208

LUNCH:

1 small carrot and 1 large celery stalk	30
1 cup plain, low-fat yogurt	130
1 sliced small banana	85
5 saltine crackers	60
Iced tea	0
	305

DINNER:

3/4 cup tomato juice	35
6 ounces sea bass baked with lemon and lime juice, parsley and garlic	173
3/4 cup brussels sprouts	41
1 small (5-ounce) baked potato with	106
1 tablespoon sour cream with chives	30

	Calories
1 slice whole wheat bread	65
Radish and watercress salad:	15
4 sliced radishes	
1 cup watercress	
Lemon juice or garlic wine vinegar	
Coffee or tea	0
1/2 cup fresh or frozen blueberries (unsweetened)	48
	513

SNACK:

Strawberry treat:
    Mix in a blender or food processor   142
        1 cup skim milk
        1 cup frozen strawberries (unsweetened)

TOTAL CALORIES FOR DAY = 1,168

DAY 3

	Calories
BREAKFAST:	
Apricot eye-opener:	265
2 tablespoons grapenuts cereal	
2/3 cup 100% Bran Flakes	
1/2 cup plain, low-fat yogurt (or 3/4 cup skim milk)	
5 dried apricot halves	
Coffee or tea	0
	265
LUNCH:	
California sandwich:	253
1 slice cracked wheat bread	
2 tablespoons low-fat cream cheese (Neufchatel)	
1/3 sliced cucumber (unpeeled)	
1/4 sliced avocado	
1/4 cup alfalfa sprouts	
1/2 sliced medium tomato	
1 cup skim milk	88
	341

	Calories

AFTERNOON TREAT AT DUNKIN' DONUTS:

6 yeast-raised Munchkins (2 with glaze)	176
Coffee or tea	0
	176

DINNER

3 ounces baked ham:	
glazed with 1 teaspoon frozen orange juice concentrate	173
1 small baked sweet potato	148
1 cup French-style string beans with	31
1/2 cup sliced mushrooms	5
1 small orange	49
Coffee or tea	0
	406

TOTAL CALORIES FOR DAY = 1,188

DAY 4

	Calories

BREAKFAST:

1/6 of a 5-inch cantaloupe	20
1 toasted English muffin	140
1 ounce melted Swiss cheese	105
Coffee or tea	0
	265

LUNCH:

3/4 cup low-fat cottage cheese	135
1 medium tomato, cut in wedges	33
1/2 sliced cucumber (unpeeled)	8
1 sliced small green pepper	16
2 sesame seed bread sticks	76
Coffee or tea	0
1 small apple	58
	326

DINNER:

1 cup chicken soup with rice	50

	Calories

Liver and mushrooms: — 250
  4 ounces chicken liver cooked with
  1/2 sliced onion, garlic, pepper
  10 sliced small mushrooms (fresh)
  1/4 cup chicken bouillon
  garnished with minced parsley and served on
  1 slice whole wheat toast — 65
3/4 cup cooked green beans — 35
1 cup mixed salad greens with — 20
Vinegar or lemon juice
Coffee or tea — 0
1 medium fresh peach (or 1/2 cup water-packed peach — 38
  slices)
458

SNACK:

Banana-strawberry treat: — 136
  Mix in a blender or food processor
    3/4 cup skim milk
    1/2 small banana
    1/2 cup frozen strawberries (unsweetened)

  TOTAL CALORIES FOR DAY = 1,185

DAY 5

	Calories

BREAKFAST:

1 cup Total cereal with — 108
3/4 cup skim milk and — 66
1/2 cup fresh or frozen strawberries (unsweetened) — 27
Coffee or tea — 0
201

LUNCH:

Good Earth salad: — 175
  1 cup romaine lettuce
  1/2 cup fresh spinach

	Calories

4 sliced large mushrooms (fresh)
1/4 cup alfalfa sprouts
1/4 cup kidney beans
1 sliced medium tomato
1/4 cup chick peas
Thinly sliced Bermuda onions
Vinegar or lemon juice

1 slice whole wheat bread with	65
1/2 teaspoon margarine	17
1 cup skim milk	88
	345

DINNER AT KENTUCKY FRIED CHICKEN (eaten at home):

1 piece chicken rib	199
(add 87 more calories for extra crispy)	
Cole slaw	122
Mashed potatoes and gravy	86
Roll (order it without butter)	61
Coffee or tea	0
1/6 of 5-inch cantaloupe	20
	488

SNACK:

Blueberry yogurt freeze:	132

Mix in blender or food processor
    1/2 cup frozen blueberries (unsweetened)
    1/2 small banana
    1/2 cup plain, low-fat yogurt
    Dash of cinnamon

TOTAL CALORIES FOR DAY = 1,166

DAY 6

	Calories

BREAKFAST:

3/4 cup orange juice	90
1 1/2 cups Special K cereal with	105
1 tablespoon raisins and	29
3/4 cup skim milk	66
Coffee or tea	0
	290

	Calories

LUNCH:

Special bean salad:	240
3/4 cup three-bean salad	
1/4 cup chick peas	
1/2 cubed cucumber (unpeeled)	
1/4 cup alfalfa sprouts	
2 teaspoons minced Bermuda onions	
Garlic wine vinegar	
Lettuce leaves	
1/2 cup low-fat cottage cheese	45
2 sesame seed bread sticks	76
Coffee or tea	0
1 small orange	49
	410

DINNER:

1 cup minestrone soup	90
6 ounce flounder broiled with lemon and parsley	120
1 cup cooked zucchini	22
1 cup cooked carrots	23
1 slice whole wheat bread	65
Salad:	35
1 sliced medium tomato	
Garlic wine vinegar	
Basil	
Coffee or tea	0
1 cup fresh strawberries	54
	409

SNACK:

1 cup skim milk	88

TOTAL CALORIES FOR DAY = 1,197

DAY 7

	Calories

BREAKFAST:

1/2 cup stewed prunes (unsweetened)	127
3/4 cup cooked oatmeal with	98

	Calories
1 tablespoon raisins and	29
1/2 cup skimmed milk	44
Coffee or tea	0
	298

LUNCH:

Tuna salad sandwich:	190
2 ounces tuna (water packed)	
1/2 tablespoon minced onion	
1 tablespoon chopped celery	
1 teaspoon minced parsley	
Lemon juice	
1 teaspoon mayonnaise	
1 sliced medium tomato	
Lettuce leaves	
1 slice whole-grain bread	
Iced tea	0
1/2 cup fresh grapes	53
	243

DINNER:

5 ounces broiled flank steak	250
1 grilled medium tomato	33
5 asparagus spears	26
1 cup mixed salad greens with	20
lemon juice or vinegar	
1 slice whole wheat bread	65
Coffee or tea	0
1 medium orange	73
	467

SNACK:

Raspberry treat:	169
Mix in a blender or food processor	
1 cup skim milk	
1/2 small banana	
1/2 cup frozen raspberries (unsweetened)	

TOTAL CALORIES FOR DAY = 1,177